AT MY TABLE

Allen & Unwin

83 Alexander Street
Crows Nest NSW 2065
Australia
Phone: (61 2) 8425 0100
Email: info@allenandunwin.com
Web: www.allenandunwin.com

Cataloguing-in-Publication details are available from the National Library of Australia
www.trove.nla.gov.au

ISBN 978 1 74237 731 5

NOTE: We have used Australian cup measures, of 250 ml (9 fl oz). Please note that the US and UK cup measures are slightly smaller, approximately 235 ml (7¾ fl oz). The nutritional analysis in each Nutrition Information Panel (NIP), unless stated otherwise, is based on one serve.

IMPORTANT: Those who might be at risk from the effects of salmonella poisoning (the elderly, pregnant women, young children and those suffering from immune deficiency diseases) should consult their doctor with any concerns about eating raw eggs.

OVEN GUIDE: You may find cooking times vary depending on the oven you are using. For fan-forced ovens, as a general rule, set the oven temperature to 20°C (35°F) lower than indicated in the recipe.

MEASURES GUIDE: We have used 20 ml (4 teaspoon) tablespoon measures. If you are using a 15 ml (3 teaspoon) tablespoon add an extra teaspoon of the ingredient for each tablespoon specified.

Set in 10.5/14 pt Rockwell by Seymour Designs

All photographs by Greg Elms Photography, except for the following: pages 25 and 64, Luke Burgess; page 50, Franz Scheurer; page 72, Dean Cambray; and page 127, Mark Chew. Recipe on page 73, from *Your Place or Mine?* by Gary Mehigan and George Calombaris, and recipe on page 126, from *Comfort Food* by Gary Mehigan, both published by Penguin/ Lantern, Melbourne, 2010, and reproduced with permission by Penguin Group (Australia).

Colour reproduction by Megan Ellis.

Printed in China by C & C Offset Printing Co., Ltd.

10 9 8 7 6 5 4 3 2 1

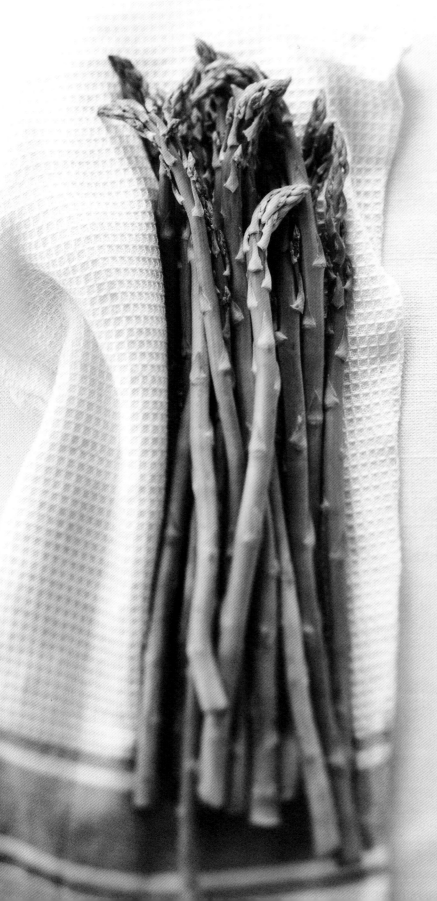

AT MY TABLE

Delicious recipes from
60 celebrated chefs for
people with diabetes

EDITED BY
AMANDA BILSON
AND JANNI KYRITSIS

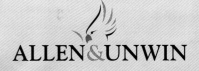

ALLEN&UNWIN

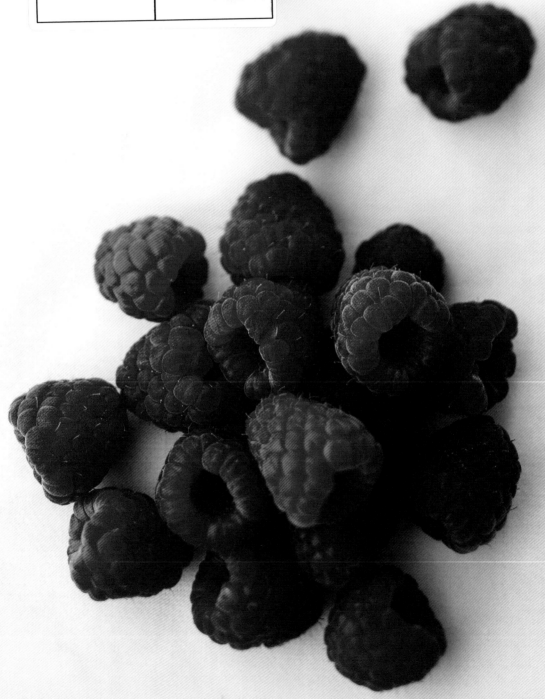

FOREWORD

The idea for this cookbook was not to make it 'diabetes friendly' in the traditional sense, but to make it 'consumer friendly' by including the basic nutrition information for each recipe and a little dietitian tip for guidance for anyone who may be watching their weight, blood glucose levels or cholesterol. We would never presume to ask these wonderful chefs to alter their recipes in any way, but you may see that sometimes I have suggested alternative ingredients or different preparation tips if you wish to make a change. I emphasise that any suggested changes may mean a change in flavour and/or texture to the recipe, so don't blame the chef – blame me.

The money raised from the sales of this cookbook will go directly towards funding services provided by the staff for patients, their families and carers at the St Vincent's Hospital Diabetes Centre. We are still going strong after 31 years but we need your help to continue our work as several of our staff members are supported by these types of fundraising efforts.

I would like to thank my colleague Kylie Alexander for her meticulous work with the nutritional anlaysis of the recipes. On behalf of Kylie and myself, I would also like to send a big thank you to Eileen, Janni and Amanda for the hard work, effort and enthusiasm that they have provided for this project. Finally, thank you to all our contributing chefs who have given very freely of their recipes and have found time to answer all our little questions and queries over the past several months. They are the undisputed stars of this book.

Happy cooking and consuming.

Melissa Armstrong AdvAPD, CDE
Senior Clinical Dietitian

 The Diabetes Centre, St Vincent's Hospital

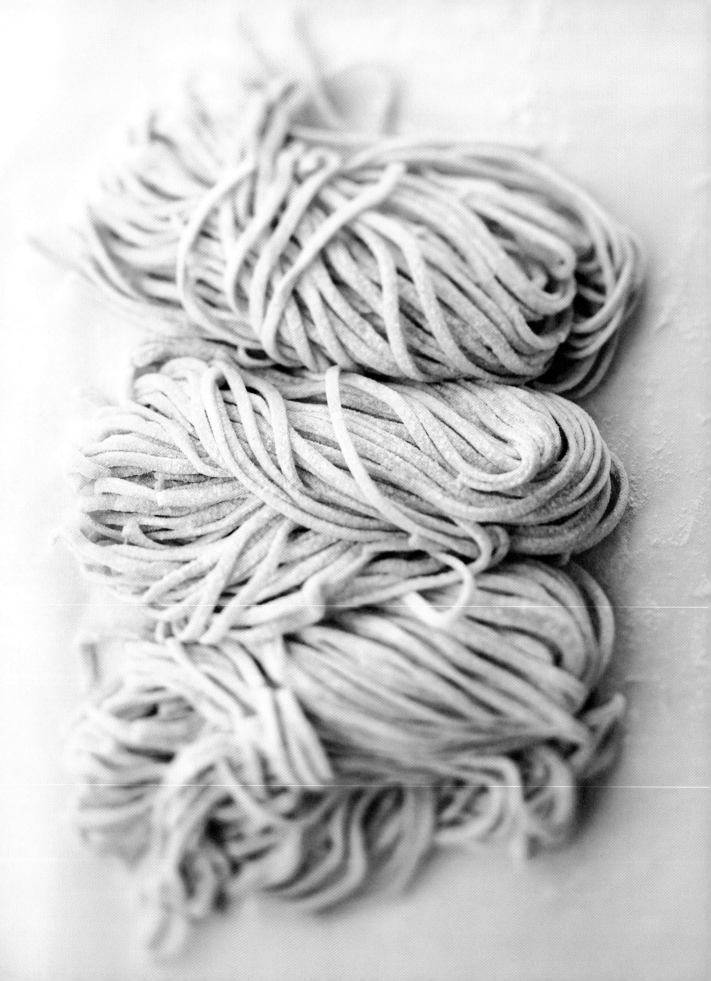

CONTENTS

FOREWORD V

INTRODUCTION BY
AMANDA BILSON AND JANNI KYRITSIS IX

ENTRÉES 1

SEAFOOD 45

MEAT 85

VEGETABLES, SALADS AND PASTA 133

DESSERTS 167

CONTRIBUTORS' BIOGRAPHIES 205

INDEX 215

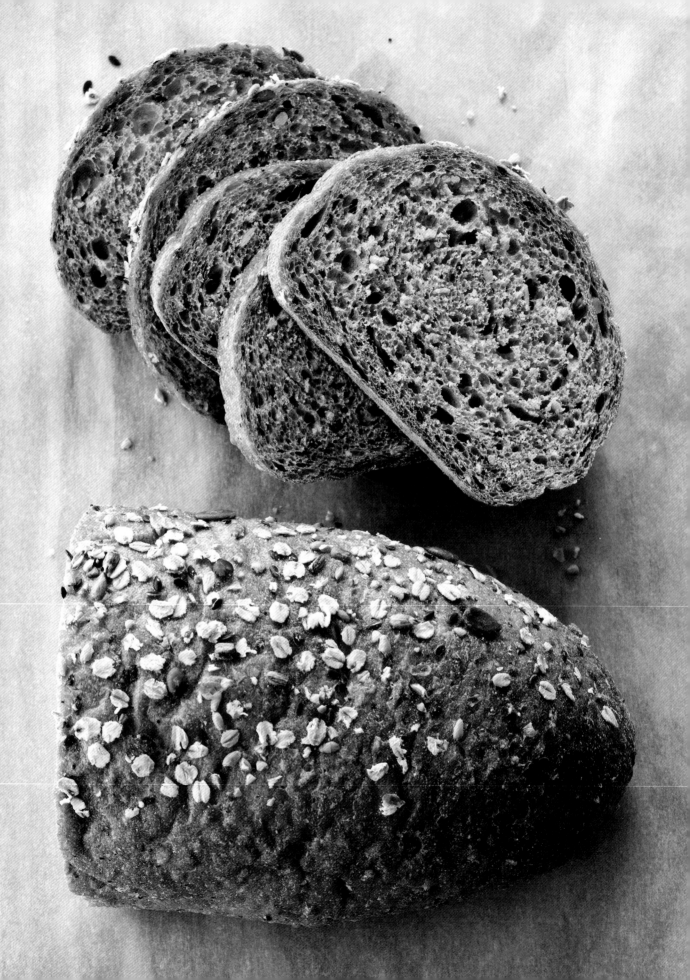

INTRODUCTION

AMANDA BILSON

I grew up in England in a large, happy family as the fourth of six children. I had a healthy, active childhood and was a very keen ballet dancer. But at age 15, just after I moved to a new school to start studying for my A levels, I suddenly developed an insatiable thirst together with a strange lethargy and an inability to concentrate. I would get home from school and literally collapse with exhaustion and a terrible aching in my legs.

The symptoms didn't last too long before Mum took me to our local GP. He did a urine test, whereupon I was rushed to the local hospital. There I was diagnosed with Type 1 diabetes. I was admitted for two weeks in order to stabilise my blood sugars, learn how to inject insulin and understand what I could and couldn't eat. I was sent home with a lot of cumbersome paraphernalia and the prospect of a rather terrifying future.

This was the start of my new life with Type 1 diabetes, and it has been a journey of lifelong learning – about diet, food values, maintaining balance and the value of exercise. Ultimately it's about constant management and never letting it get you down. In fact the most important lesson I have learned is that living with diabetes is about making it your friend, not your enemy.

In 1984 I left London and a successful career in publishing to start a new life in Sydney. I met famous chef Tony Bilson in 1985 and we fell in love, married and had two beautiful children. They have had to learn about diabetes too, and managing Mum when she's having a hypo has not always been easy!

Now, 45 years since my condition was first diagnosed, I am proud to say that diabetes has never prevented me from living a full and exciting life. Part of the reason for that is the enormous help I have received from the dedicated professionals at the Diabetes Centre, part of St Vincent's Hospital, Sydney. The doctors, nurses, dietitians and support staff have always been there when needed, volunteering advice and support.

When Eileen Anastas, fundraising coordinator at the Centre, asked me to be involved with a book project, I was delighted, given my background in publishing. Together with Janni Kyritsis, the three of us came up with the idea of approaching our friends in the restaurant industry and asking them to donate recipes for a cookbook that anyone with diabetes in their family could enjoy using. This volume is the result and we are delighted with the range and variety of recipes included.

I would like to extend my thanks and gratitude to the talented chefs from all round Australia who have contributed to this worthy cause. I would also like to thank Kylie Alexander and Melissa Armstrong, dietitians at the Centre, who spent many hours analysing each recipe; Eileen, whose care, energy and enthusiasm made it a truly enjoyable project; and at Allen & Unwin, our publisher Annette Barlow and editor Sarah Baker, ever patient and rigorous in dealing with 60 authors and two editors!

Finally, I would like to thank my husband Tony, who has cooked me countless beautiful dishes and from whom I have learned so much.

JANNI KYRITSIS

It was a shock when I was diagnosed with Type 2 diabetes four years ago but, in my case, a wake-up call to change my life and improve my health. I love food and its preparation. It's the reason my partner David suggested 35 years ago that I give up my career as an electrician and become a chef.

Growing up in Greece, eating with family and friends was a big part of life. That enjoyment I brought with me to Australia. But one has to learn moderation and, as a chef, moderation was not part of my vocabulary. My life was dedicated to creating and, of course, tasting new dishes along with eating out and enjoying every occasion. I didn't stop to think about the consequences of such a lifestyle on my health.

It was soon after hanging up my chef's hat at my MG Garage restaurant that the diagnosis was made. Dealing with the prospect of a health condition that would be with me for the rest of my life was daunting. Thanks to the care and attention I received at the Diabetes Centre I felt empowered to take action and deal with this diagnosis with a positive approach.

To my surprise, once I started considering my diet more carefully, I managed to lose 20 kilograms. I did not really go on an elaborate diet or deprive myself of food; I just became sensible and stopped eating those rich desserts. No more raiding the fridge at 1 am to see what sweets I could find. I also started to exercise, and realised that I hadn't felt so good for years.

During one of my many visits to the Diabetes Centre I met Eileen Anastas, who coordinates fundraising at the Centre. She told me she had been a regular customer of mine, following me from Berowra Waters Inn to Bennelong and then MG Garage. She was very happy to hear that I had retired, and immediately urged me to help with a project that she wanted to get off the ground – producing a cookbook. As well as raising funds for patient programs at the Diabetes Centre, Eileen wanted a book that offered more freedom of choice for people with diabetes, more choice balanced with moderation.

We then approached Amanda Bilson, another patient of the Diabetes Centre, so that we could develop this project. Not only did Amanda agree to help but, after our first meeting, she came up with the idea of a celebrity chef cookbook and also agreed to take on the daunting role of editor. Between us, Amanda and I were able to call on our many friends in the food industry to contribute recipes. We asked chefs to provide recipes that didn't need great professional skills, but enough skill to stretch one's creativity. A love of preparing good food was an essential ingredient.

I have created most of the dessert recipes with an emphasis on light. I know that desserts can be a stumbling block for cooks and I hope you will be pleasantly surprised at how simple it can be to produce a delicious sweet dish. Don't expect culinary masterpieces such as puff pastry, super rich brioche, feather light soufflés and the smoother ice creams. Instead you will find granitas, jellies and chocolate mousse with a twist, for a bit of indulgence. These are very easy recipes with ingredients that can be found in any grocers and/or greengrocers.

Amanda, Eileen and I are very grateful for the generosity of all the chefs who have kindly taken time to participate in this most worthwhile project. We couldn't be more delighted with the fantastic recipes. All that is left is for you to enjoy cooking these recipes for your family and friends.

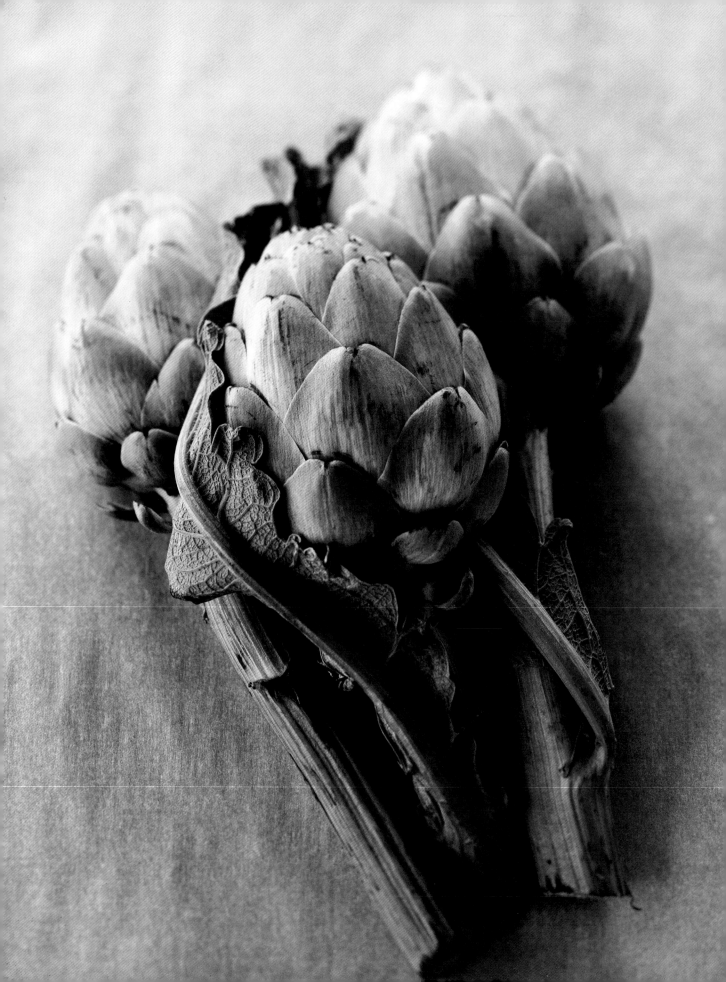

ENTRÉES

MUSHROOM SOUP WITH PORCINI

STEPHANIE ALEXANDER

This recipe is based on one in my book *Kitchen Garden Companion*. It is a rustic soup, woodsy in colour and flavour. Dried porcini mushrooms are sold in small envelopes in larger supermarkets and specialty food stores. They need preliminary soaking.

1 cup (250 ml/9 fl oz) boiling water

15 g (½ oz) dried porcini mushrooms

500 g (1 lb 2 oz) mushrooms (see note)

40 g (1½ oz) butter

1 onion, sliced

2 garlic cloves, chopped

2 tsp thyme leaves

1 tbsp chopped flat-leaf (Italian) parsley

1 thick slice sourdough bread, cut into 2-cm (¾-in) cubes

4 cups (1 litre/35 fl oz) chicken stock, vegetable stock or water

2 tbsp tomato paste (concentrated purée)

sea salt and freshly ground pepper

OPTIONAL GARNISH

2 tbsp commercial horseradish cream, pressed to remove as much vinegar as possible, then mixed with the same quantity of thin (pouring) cream

SERVES 6

Pour boiling water over porcini and soak for 15 minutes. Lift porcini from liquid and chop roughly, then set aside. Strain soaking liquid through a fine sieve and reserve. Coarsely chop fresh mushrooms in a food processor.

Melt butter in a large saucepan over medium heat, then cook onion for 5 minutes, or until it starts to soften. Add garlic, thyme, parsley and chopped porcini and sauté for 1 minute, then tip in strained porcini juice. Bring to the boil. Add chopped mushrooms, bread, stock or water and tomato paste. Stir and bring to simmering point. Taste and add salt and pepper. Reduce heat to low and simmer for 10 minutes.

Blend soup in a food processor until quite smooth. Adjust seasoning. If soup is too thick, add a little hot water.

Serve in heated soup bowls, with a dollop of horseradish cream, if using.

NOTE: You can use buttons or flats, regular mushrooms or Swiss browns, or a mixture.

DIETITIAN TIP
A low-fat and low-carbohydrate choice.

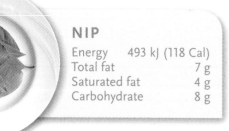

NIP

Energy	493 kJ (118 Cal)
Total fat	7 g
Saturated fat	4 g
Carbohydrate	8 g

STEAMED OYSTERS WITH KAFFIR LIME LEAF, CHILLI AND GINGER

STEVEN SNOW

Great for parties and as a cocktail canapé.

12 Sydney rock or Pacific oysters, freshly shucked

1 kaffir lime leaf, thinly sliced

1 small knob ginger, thinly sliced

1 red banana chilli, seeds removed and finely chopped

25 ml (1 fl oz) tamari or light soy sauce

squeeze of lime juice

SERVES 2 AS AN ENTRÉE

Place oysters in a 25-cm (10-in) bamboo steamer basket. Top each oyster with kaffir leaf, ginger and chilli. Set aside.

Heat a wok with 1 cm (½ in) of water in the base and bring to the boil. Place steamer basket with lid over boiling water, cover and steam for 1¾ minutes. Do not overcook oysters.

Pour tamari or soy sauce over oysters, squeeze on lime juice and serve immediately to make the most of the aromas.

DIETITIAN TIP
A great low-energy starter.

NIP

Energy	52 kJ (12 Cal)
Total fat	0.4 g
Saturated fat	0.1 g
Carbohydrate	NIL

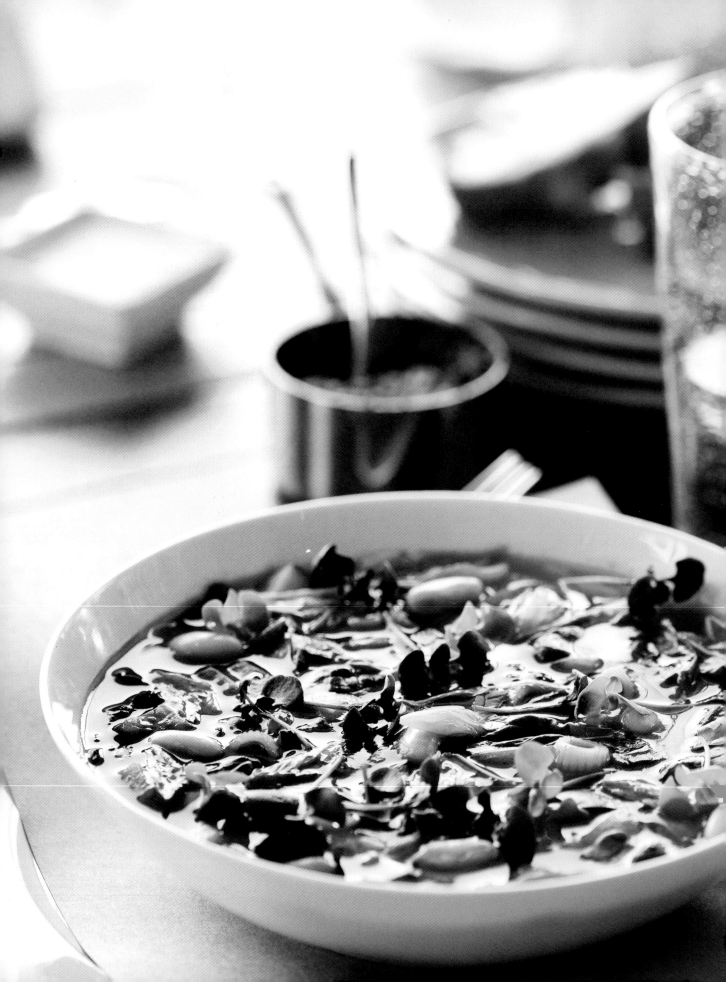

VEGETABLE MINESTRONE WITH RICOTTA PESTO

KEVIN DONOVAN

1–2 tbsp olive oil

3 onions, finely diced

2 celery stalks, finely diced

1 handful flat-leaf (Italian) parsley leaves

6 cups (1.5 litres/52 fl oz) vegetable stock

2 potatoes, cut into 1-cm (½-in) cubes

8 roma (plum) tomatoes, peeled, seeds removed and diced

½–1 zucchini (courgette), cut into 1-cm (½-in) cubes

⅓ cup (50 g/1¾ oz) fresh peas

50 g (1¾ oz) green beans, cut into 2-cm (¾-in) lengths

50 g (1¾ oz) tinned drained borlotti beans

4 silverbeet (Swiss chard) leaves, stalks removed and discarded, leaves chopped

1 cup (175 g/6 oz) cooked rigatoni

sea salt and freshly ground pepper

ricotta cheese, for crumbling over soup

RICOTTA PESTO

1 garlic clove

2 tsp pine nuts

1 tbsp freshly grated parmesan cheese

50 g (1¾ oz) ricotta cheese

2½ tbsp olive oil

2 cups basil, leaves only

MAKES 2 LITRES (70 FL OZ) / SERVES 8

Heat olive oil in a large saucepan over medium heat. Add onion, celery and parsley and cook until soft but without colour. Add vegetable stock, potato and tomato and bring to the boil, then simmer for 20 minutes until soft. Add zucchini, peas and green beans and cook soup for a further 15 minutes until vegetables are soft but still retain their shape. Remove from heat and strain into another large saucepan, reserving vegetables. Return half the cooked vegetables to the soup and blend with a hand-held blender until puréed. Return remaining vegetables to soup.

Return pan to heat and add borlotti beans, silverbeet and rigatoni. Simmer for 5 minutes.

For ricotta pesto, blend all ingredients except basil in a food processor until smooth. Add basil and blend until smooth.

To serve, stir 4 tablespoons pesto into soup. Add salt and pepper to taste and ladle into warm bowls. Garnish with crumbled ricotta.

DIETITIAN TIP
A terrific high-fibre entrée choice.

NIP

Energy	869 kJ (208 Cal)
Total fat	12 g
Saturated fat	2 g
Carbohydrate	16 g

CRAB BOUDIN IN A COMPOSED SALAD

CHUI LEE LUK

This is a play on the traditional *boudin blanc*.

EGGPLANT CUSTARD

2 Japanese eggplants (aubergines)

3½ tbsp olive oil

1½ tbsp Champagne, plus extra to taste

1 tbsp mirin, plus extra to taste

sea salt and freshly ground white pepper

1 × 60 g (2¼ oz) egg

CRAB BOUDIN

1 kg (2 lb 4 oz) freshly picked raw spanner crabmeat

2 eggs

100 ml (3½ fl oz) chicken stock

dry vermouth

sea salt and freshly ground white pepper

AVOCADO DRESSING

100 ml (3½ fl oz) chicken stock

1 tbsp glutinous rice wine

½ avocado

sea salt and freshly ground white pepper

SALAD

spring onion (scallion) sprouts
(3 or 4 per person)

salad burnet leaf (4 leaves per person)

grilled (broiled) asparagus spears
(2 spears per person)

SERVES 4

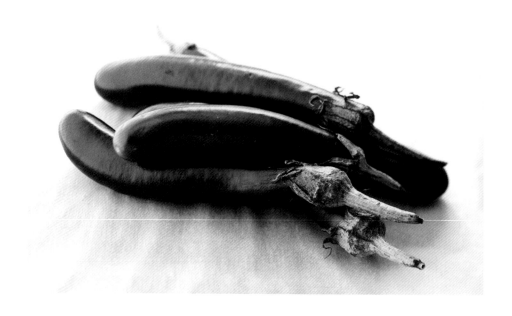

Preheat oven to 200°C (400°F/Gas 6).

For eggplant custard, first make eggplant purée by frying whole eggplants in an oven-proof frying pan with 1 tablespoon olive oil over medium heat until golden brown. Finish in oven until cooked through, about 5–10 minutes. Press to remove excess oil and moisture, then drain while letting them cool. Purée and pass through a sieve. Season mixture with Champagne, mirin to add sweetness, salt and white pepper. Beat egg and pass through a sieve to ensure there's no foam or albumen. Combine with eggplant purée. It is important to pay attention to the proportion of egg, eggplant purée and Champagne to ensure the mixture sets. Season with extra Champagne, remaining olive oil, extra mirin, salt and white pepper.

Place half a tablespoonful of eggplant purée on a 33 × 33-cm (13 × 13-in) piece of plastic wrap, enclose and twist top to form a little ball, tie with kitchen twine or twist plastic into a knot. The purée should make about 8 balls, depending on the size of each one. Drop into a saucepan of water just below simmering point and poach for 5 minutes until set. Unwrap, ready to place onto the salad arrangement with the crab boudin when required.

Crab boudin is best made in large quantities; any excess can be stored in the freezer. Process crabmeat with eggs in a food processor until it is a thick white mass that holds its shape, then fold through chicken stock. Season with vermouth, salt and white pepper. Again, place half tablespoonfuls on pieces of plastic wrap, twist the ends to enclose the crab mixture and shape into balls. (You will need 8 balls.) Poach in a saucepan of water to just below simmering point for approximately 5 minutes.

Prick one of the balls with a skewer. If it is done, nothing will ooze out. Unwrap the balls and refresh in iced water until chilled through. Remove and set aside until ready to use.

For avocado dressing, mix chicken stock with rice wine, then purée with avocado. Season with salt and pepper. This must be used within a couple of hours otherwise it will oxidise and go brown.

To assemble, put two each of the crab balls and eggplant balls on each piece of crispy choux pastry (see page 8). Place spoonfuls of avocado dressing around the plate in an attractive manner, then scatter over the salad garnish.

CHOUX PASTRY

This recipe yields 1 kg (2 lb 4 oz) choux pastry, more than is required, so use excess pastry to make éclairs etc., if desired, or cook until crisp and use as crisp breads.

1 cup (250 ml/9 fl oz) milk

1 cup (250 ml/9 fl oz) water

200 g (7 oz) butter

1 tsp salt

1½ tbsp sugar

2 cups (300 g/10½ oz) plain (all-purpose) flour, sifted

8 eggs

Preheat oven to 210°C (415°F/Gas 6–7). Line a baking tray with baking paper.

Bring milk, water, butter, salt and sugar to the boil in a saucepan. Add flour away from heat, stirring well. Return to low heat and cook, stirring constantly, until mixture comes away from side of pan, about 5 minutes. Turn mixture out into the bowl of an electric mixer and start whisking. Add eggs one at a time, beating well after each addition. Resulting mixture should be thick and sticking to side of bowl.

Spread tablespoonfuls of choux mixture out to 2 mm (1/16 in) thick in attractive shapes on baking trays. Bake for 6 minutes, reduce oven temperature to 180°C (350°F/Gas 4) and bake for another 6 minutes, then reduce temperature to 150°C (300°F/Gas 2) and bake for up to 15 minutes. Pastry is ready when it's dried and crisped. These baking times depend on your oven, so if pastry's too dark, reduce temperature on third reduction so that pastry has a chance to dry out and not colour further.

DIETITIAN TIP
Great for a dinner party, rather than as an everyday food.

NIP
Energy	2522 kJ (603 Cal)
Total fat	38 g
Saturated fat	12 g
Carbohydrate	15 g

SCALLOPS WITH GREEN OLIVE TAPENADE AND PRESERVED LEMON POWDER

ADAM LIAW

1 preserved lemon

12 scallops, on their shells, roe removed

1 tbsp olive oil

sea salt

1 tbsp hazelnut oil

GREEN OLIVE TAPENADE

½ cup (90 g/3¼ oz) green olives

1 tsp lemon juice

1 tbsp finely chopped flat-leaf (Italian) parsley

SERVES 4

To make green olive tapenade, soak olives in cold water in fridge overnight then pit them. Add olive flesh to a food processor and pulse till it achieves a chunky tapenade-like consistency. Stir through lemon juice and parsley.

Preheat oven to 60°C (140°F/Gas ¼).

Remove and discard pith, flesh and seeds from preserved lemon and cut zest into julienne. Spread zest on a sheet of baking paper and bake for about 4 hours until it is dry and brittle. Grind using a mortar and pestle to a fine powder.

Brush scallops with a little olive oil, season and fry them in a very hot frying pan over high heat for 30 seconds on each side. They should be just browned but still translucent in the centre. Remove from pan and brush with a little hazelnut oil.

Sterilise scallop shells by boiling them in water, then dry them. Add a little olive tapenade to each shell and top with a scallop, then sprinkle over preserved lemon powder.

DIETITIAN TIP
A low-carbohydrate and low-fat choice.

NIP

Energy	608 kJ (145 Cal)
Total fat	11 g
Saturated fat	2 g
Carbohydrate	2 g

A TAPAS RECIPE – WHITE ANCHOVIES WITH CAPERBERRIES AND ROASTED ONION

LAUREN MURDOCH

2 red (Spanish) onions, cut into large wedges

2 tbsp extra virgin olive oil

sea salt and freshly ground pepper

1 tsp sherry vinegar

32 large white anchovy fillets

24 caperberries

8 tbsp roughly chopped flat-leaf (Italian) parsley

4 tbsp roughly chopped mint

zest of ½ lemon

crusty bread, to serve

SERVES 4

Preheat oven to 200°C (400°F/Gas 6).

Drizzle onion with a little olive oil, season and roast in oven for about 15–20 minutes.

Toss roasted onion in vinegar and set aside to cool.

Gently toss together onion and remaining ingredients then serve with crusty bread.

DIETITIAN TIP
A recipe with a high proportion of the fat as omega 3.

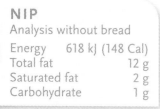

NIP
Analysis without bread

Energy	618 kJ (148 Cal)
Total fat	12 g
Saturated fat	2 g
Carbohydrate	1 g

SEARED SCALLOPS WITH CAULIFLOWER PURÉE, SHIITAKE MUSHROOMS AND VEAL JUS

GUILLAUME BRAHIMI

6 cups (1.5 litres/52 fl oz) chicken stock

1 kg (2 lb 4 oz) cauliflower florets

180 ml (6 fl oz) thin (pouring) cream

40 g (1½ oz) butter

100 g (3½ oz) shiitake mushrooms, stalks removed, caps quartered

sea salt and freshly ground pepper

18 large scallops

½ bunch flat-leaf (Italian) parsley, finely chopped

VEAL JUS

500 g (1 lb 2 oz) veal osso buco

MIREPOIX

½ garlic bulb

2 tomatoes

6 white peppercorns, crushed

SERVES 6

For veal jus, brown off veal pieces and mirepoix ingredients in a saucepan over high heat until golden. Add to a large saucepan, cover with cold water, bring to the boil, then reduce heat to low and simmer, skimming continuously for 4–6 hours. Strain, remove and discard all fat, veal bones and mirepoix, then return stock to a saucepan and cook over medium–high heat until it has a sauce-like consistency and has reduced to 1 cup (250 ml/9 fl oz).

In a large saucepan, bring chicken stock to the boil, add cauliflower, reduce heat to low, cover and simmer until tender, about 15 minutes. Strain cauliflower into a blender, purée and return to pan.

Whip cream and add slowly to puréed cauliflower until combined. Set aside.

In a frying pan over high heat, melt butter and pan-fry mushrooms until golden brown. Season with salt and pepper, remove from pan and set aside.

Seal scallops in a frying pan over medium–high heat for 45 seconds before turning and cooking for another 10 seconds.

To serve, pour cauliflower purée onto each serving plate and top with mushrooms. Place scallops evenly around purée, pour 2 tablespoons veal jus onto each plate and sprinkle with parsley.

DIETITIAN TIP

The cream and butter make this recipe higher in saturated fat than some of the others so, if your cholesterol is high, beware.

NIP

Energy	1029 kJ (246 Cal)
Total fat	18 g
Saturated fat	10 g
Carbohydrate	7 g

SASHIMI YELLOW FIN TUNA SPRING ROLLS WITH EDAMAME SAUCE

DAMIAN HEADS

4 large savoy cabbage leaves

4 × 80 g (2¾ oz) strips sashimi tuna (see note, page 14)

freshly ground black pepper

pickled ginger

1 tbsp plain (all-purpose) flour

approximately 2 tbsp water

4 spring roll wrappers

700 ml (24 fl oz) vegetable oil, for frying

SERVES 4

EDAMAME SAUCE

250 g (9 oz) frozen edamame (green soya beans)

½ long green chilli, split and seeds removed

4 stems coriander (cilantro), leaves picked

2½ tbsp extra virgin olive oil

juice of 1 lime

sea salt

GARNISH

100 g (3½ oz) frozen edamame, thawed and soya beans removed from pod

salt-reduced soy sauce

green Tabasco sauce

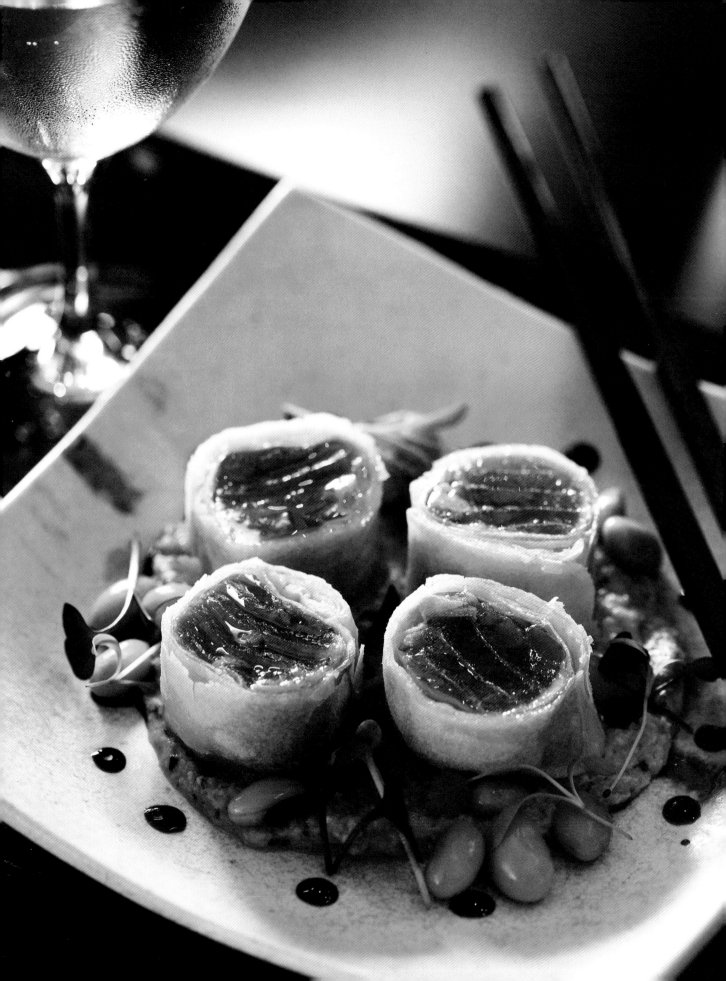

For spring rolls, blanch cabbage leaves in a large saucepan of salted boiling water for 2 minutes, refresh them in iced water before draining and pressing dry in a clean tea towel. Cut off thick stems from cabbage leaves.

Lay out cabbage pieces on a work surface. Place a piece of sashimi tuna on each (but if cabbage seems excessive, trim it, as desired result is to wrap tuna once with just a slight overlap – the ends don't need to be wrapped). Season tuna with a turn of cracked black pepper then arrange a single layer of pickled ginger on top. Roll cabbage tightly around tuna and ginger.

Mix flour with enough water to make a thin batter.

Use one spring roll wrapper at a time and place on a clean bench. Place a cabbage roll towards bottom of wrapper. Fold sides in and then roll up, keeping it as tight as possible. Brush batter on end of wrapper to seal it. Place finished rolls on paper towel in fridge, overnight at the most.

For edamame sauce, place edamame in a small saucepan with enough water to cover. Place the pan over medium heat and bring to a simmer, then remove from heat. Drain the cooking liquor, reserving ½ cup (125 ml/4 fl oz). Remove soya beans from their pods while warm. Place soya beans in bowl of a food processor with reserved liquor, chilli, coriander and olive oil. Blend to a sauce (slightly lumpy is okay). Add lime juice and enough salt to enhance flavour of finished sauce.

Heat vegetable oil to 180°C (350°F) in a deep-fryer or 3-litre(105-fl oz) saucepan (there must be no risk of oil boiling over). Place one spring roll at a time in hot oil and fry for 45 seconds. Remove spring roll with a slotted spoon and drain on paper towel. Repeat frying process with remaining three rolls.

Lightly trim ends from each roll, then cut each into four pieces. Place a dollop of edamame sauce in centre of each serving plate, then arrange four pieces of spring roll, cut side up, on top. Garnish with some scattered soya beans, a drizzle of soy sauce and green Tabasco sauce on each slice.

NOTE: Buy a 500-g (1 lb 2-oz) piece of sashimi grade tuna. Cut four even strips from it and use any trimmings for a tataki dish. (If you can't get good tuna, sashimi salmon would be a good alternative.)

DIETITIAN TIP
Tuna is a great source of the essential omega 3 fats.

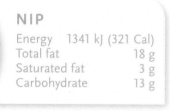

NIP
Energy   1341 kJ (321 Cal)
Total fat   18 g
Saturated fat   3 g
Carbohydrate   13 g

SEA SCALLOP CEVICHE

CHRISTINE MANFIELD

16 large Hervey Bay scallops, trimmed

MARINADE

1 ruby grapefruit, peeled and sliced
into segments

2½ tbsp lime juice

2½ tbsp ruby grapefruit juice

1½ tbsp orange juice

1 tsp sea salt (Fleur de Sel)

1½ tbsp sugar syrup

2 tbsp shredded mint leaves

2 red Asian shallots, finely diced

1 small green chilli, minced

GARNISH

2 tbsp snipped chives

2 tbsp celery cress

4 thin slices prosciutto, grilled (broiled)
till crisp then crumbled

SERVES 4

Slice scallops into thin rounds.

Cut grapefruit segments into small dice.

Mix diced grapefruit with lime, grapefruit
and orange juices, salt and sugar syrup. Add
scallops and marinate for 15 minutes. Add mint,
shallot and chilli and mix.

Arrange scallops on serving plates, pour
over marinade dressing and sprinkle with
chives, celery cress and prosciutto crumbs.

DIETITIAN TIP

A modest serve of carbohydrate in this dish
comes from the slightly sweet dressing. To
reduce the sugar, replace with an artificial
sweetener if you wish.

NIP

Energy	650 kJ (155 Cal)
Total fat	4 g
Saturated fat	1 g
Carbohydrate	12 g

CECINA

GEORGE POMPEI

*Delicious on its own or as an accompaniment to antipasti, cecina
is a quick unleavened flatbread made with besan (chickpea flour).
The name 'cecina' refers to ceci, the Italian name for chickpeas.*

5 cups (600 g/1 lb 5 oz) besan
(chickpea flour)

8 cups (2 litres/70 fl oz) water

90 ml (3 fl oz) extra virgin olive oil

freshly ground black pepper

SERVES 8

Preheat oven to 200°C (400°F/Gas 6).

In a large bowl, gently mix besan with water
until well combined, about 5 minutes. Add oil
and mix for another minute. Pour into a shallow
baking tin so that the mixture is about 5 mm
(¼ in) high. Place in oven for 10 minutes, or
until a light golden crust forms. Add pepper
and serve immediately.

DIETITIAN TIP
Fantastically high in fibre due to the use of besan.
A great accompaniment to many of the entrées in
this section.

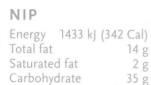

NIP
Energy   1433 kJ (342 Cal)
Total fat   14 g
Saturated fat   2 g
Carbohydrate   35 g

SALAD OF RED MULLET, SOUTHERN CALAMARI, EGGPLANT, TOMATO AND MINT

JONATHAN BARTHELMESS

4 ×125 g (4½ oz) red mullet fillets, skin on

sea salt

zest of 1 lemon

1 eggplant (aubergine)

500 g (1 lb 2 oz) ripe, flavoursome tomatoes

juice of ½ lemon

1 large green chilli, seeds removed, finely chopped

1 garlic clove, minced

1 handful mint leaves, roughly chopped

freshly ground pepper

extra virgin olive oil

250 g (9 oz) cleaned sashimi-grade calamari, shaved as finely as possible

SERVES 4

Place red mullet fillets, skin side down, on baking paper and sprinkle with pinch of salt and lemon zest and leave for 2 hours in fridge – this will start to cure and firm up the flesh.

Cut eggplant lengthways into 5-mm (¼-in) slices, sprinkle with salt, place in a colander and set aside for 1 hour.

Peel and seed tomatoes, making sure to keep all their juice, and chop roughly into 1-cm (½-in) pieces.

Place tomato in a bowl, add lemon juice, chilli, garlic and mint. Season, add 3 tablespoons extra virgin olive oil and allow to sit for 1 hour.

Use paper towel to wipe lemon zest and salt off fish fillets. Bring enough oil to cover fillets up to 45°C (115°F) in a saucepan over low heat. Add fish and cook until flesh starts to flake when you press it, about 20 minutes. Fish will appear raw but texture will be cooked. Low temperature cooking sets protein in fish without changing colour.

Meanwhile, use paper towel to wipe salt off eggplant slices. Heat a frying pan over medium heat, add ½ cup (125 ml/4 fl oz) extra virgin olive oil and fry eggplant in batches until golden brown and crisp. Remove eggplant from oil and place on paper towel. Season and allow to cool.

Heat another ½ cup (125 ml/4 fl oz) extra virgin olive oil in a large pan over high heat until oil ripples, add one-quarter of the shaved calamari and cook, moving constantly, until calamari turns white, about 15 seconds. As soon as calamari is cooked, remove from pan, place on paper towel and season. Repeat with the remaining calamari.

To serve, put 3 slices of eggplant on each plate, then a quarter of the calamari and 1 red mullet fillet. Drizzle on tomato salsa. This dish is to be served at room temperature.

DIETITIAN TIP
The fat in this recipe is mostly mono-unsaturated – a better choice for those with diabetes.

NIP

Energy	1964 kJ (469 Cal)
Total fat	38 g
Saturated fat	7 g
Carbohydrate	5 g

SALAD OF BLUE SWIMMER CRAB, HEART OF PALM, CORIANDER AND MINT

PETER DOYLE

450 g (1 lb) freshly picked blue swimmer crabmeat

1½ tbsp lemon juice

150 ml (5 fl oz) extra virgin olive oil

sea salt and freshly ground pepper

1 telegraph (long) cucumber, peeled, seeds removed, finely diced

10 coriander (cilantro) leaves, chopped

10 mint leaves, chopped

2½ tbsp Vietnamese dipping sauce

2 avocados, sliced

20 ruby grapefruit segments

20 slices heart of palm from the trimmed and peeled base end of the palm heart

30 round slices heart of palm from the smaller top end of peeled heart of palm (see note)

coriander (cilantro) cress

SERVES 10

Divide crabmeat into 10 portions.

Make a lemon vinaigrette with the lemon juice and olive oil, season with salt and pepper. Taste to make sure it is not too acidic.

Toss each portion of crabmeat in a small bowl with a little cucumber dice, chopped coriander and mint, and 1 teaspoon dipping sauce. On each serving plate, place crab mixture on top of avocado and between grapefruit segments and heart of palm slices (2 from the base end and 3 from the top end). Repeat with remaining portions. Decorate each crab salad with coriander cress and finish with lemon vinaigrette. Serve immediately.

NOTE: The opposite ends of heart of palm are quite different in appearance and yield different results.

DIETITIAN TIP
This could be served as a light meal accompanied by rye or wholemeal sourdough bread.

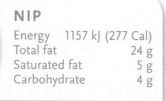

NIP
Energy	1157 kJ (277 Cal)
Total fat	24 g
Saturated fat	5 g
Carbohydrate	4 g

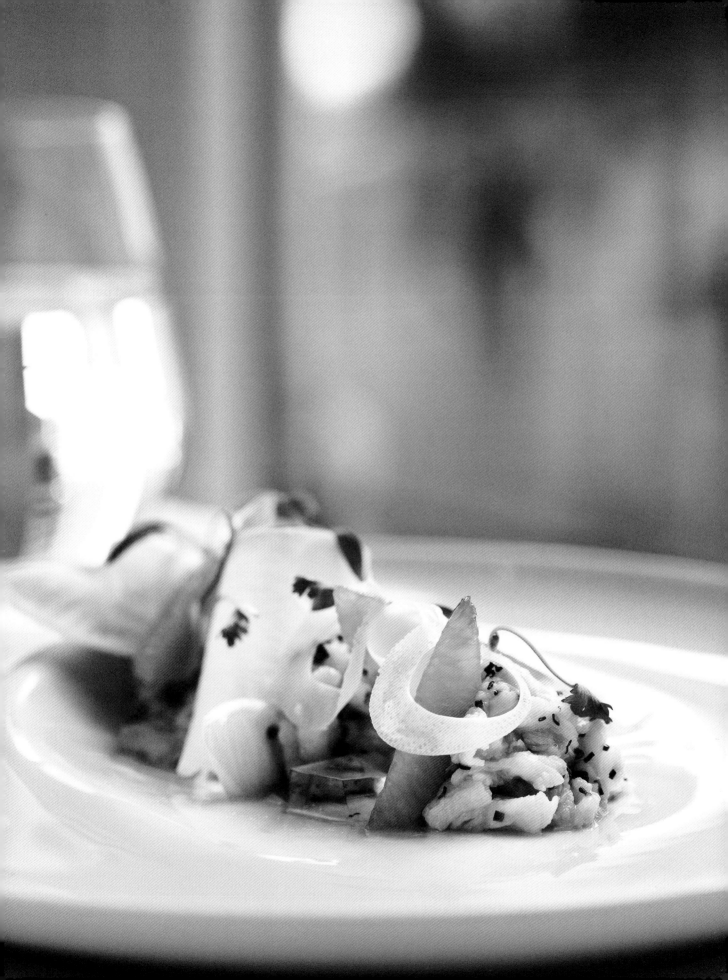

SASHIMI OF HIRAMASA KINGFISH, RAW CHINESE ARTICHOKES, PICKLED KOHLRABI, HORSERADISH

PETER GILMORE

Chinese artichokes are sometimes available at farmers' markets but are hard to come by. In Europe they are referred to as 'crones'. The best substitute would be sliced water chestnuts.

20 g (¾ oz) freshly grated horseradish

200 ml (7 fl oz) crème fraîche

sea salt

8 white celery stalks, cut into fine julienne

⅔ cup (50 g/1¾ oz) caster (superfine) sugar

200 ml (7 fl oz) good-quality apple cider vinegar

2 kohlrabi

50 g (1¾ oz) smoked eel, thinly sliced

2 cups (500 ml/17 fl oz) chicken stock

100 g (3½ oz) tapioca pearls

1 × 500 g (1 lb 2 oz) octopus

1 kg (2 lb 4 oz) hiramasa kingfish fillet, skin removed

200 ml (7 fl oz) white soy sauce

32 Chinese artichokes, cleaned

32 small nasturtium leaves

GINGER-INFUSED OIL

2 cups (500 ml/17 fl oz) grapeseed oil

40 g (1½ oz) sliced spring onions (scallions)

20 g (¾ oz) sliced fresh ginger

SERVES 8

For ginger-infused oil, warm oil and infuse spring onions and ginger for 1 hour. Strain and it's ready to use.

Fold horseradish through crème fraîche and season to taste. Set aside.

Lightly salt celery and allow to marinate for 1 hour. Rinse celery in cold water. Divide celery into 16 small bunches. Twist each bunch into a spiral and put aside.

Dissolve sugar in vinegar. Peel kohlrabi and slice on a mandoline to a thickness of 1 mm (¹⁄₃₂ in). Cut slices into 2-cm (¾-in) wide strips. Place strips in vinegar mixture and allow to marinate for 1 hour.

Combine smoked eel and chicken stock in a saucepan and bring to the boil. Turn down heat and allow to simmer gently for 10 minutes. Strain stock and discard eel. Place stock in a clean saucepan. Bring stock back to the boil and add tapioca. Stir well and cook for 7–8 minutes, or until starch in tapioca has reduced to a very small dot. Test tapioca by tasting; it should be soft but not mushy. Strain tapioca and discard stock. Place tapioca on a tray, season with salt and 1 tablespoon of ginger-infused oil. Allow tapioca to cool. When cool, form tapioca into small bundles. You will need approximately 40 bundles.

To prepare octopus, remove tentacles from body. You will only need tentacles for this recipe. With some coarse sea salt, scrub tentacles under running water. This will help to remove any slimy coating. Once fully rinsed, use a sharp knife to cut the suckers off the tentacles. Reserve the suckers for another purpose. Then cut tentacles into small lengths. Heat 460 ml (16 fl oz) ginger-infused oil in a small saucepan to 70°C (150°F). Poach sliced octopus tentacles for approximately 1 minute. Remove octopus and place in fridge.

Remove bloodline from kingfish fillet. Cut kingfish into 3-mm (⅛-in) thick slices across fillet. You will need 6 slices per person. Your slices will be approximately 7 cm (2¾ in) long.

Briefly marinate kingfish slices in white soy sauce, about 10 seconds. Drain and brush on remaining ginger-infused oil.

Squeeze out all liquid from pickled kohlrabi.

In base of each serving bowl, place 2 teaspoons horseradish crème fraîche. Place a small bundle of pickled kohlrabi on top, then 3 slices of marinated sashimi kingfish. Next place another 2 teaspoons horseradish crème fraîche on kingfish, another small bundle of pickled kohlrabi and then 3 slices of marinated kingfish. Garnish with octopus tentacles, Chinese artichokes, celery twists and smoked eel tapioca. Finally top with nasturtium leaves.

DIETITIAN TIP
It's not often you see tapioca these days; with the caster sugar it contributes a small amount of carbohydrate to this recipe.

NIP
Energy   1533 kJ (366 Cal)
Total fat   16 g
Saturated fat   6 g
Carbohydrate   17 g

LOW-FAT PRAWN LAKSA

LYNDEY MILAN

I love laksa but it is amazingly high in fat — and this is made even worse
as coconut milk is a saturated fat. But replace it with stock and light or reduced-fat
coconut milk and be sure to use rice noodles, rather than the higher fat wheat ones,
and you can enjoy it without guilt. Just keep up the flavour with herbs and spices.

100 g (3½ oz) dried or 200 g (7 oz) fresh rice noodles

1 tsp peanut oil

1 lemongrass stem, white part only, finely chopped

2 tbsp laksa paste

3 cups (750 ml/26 fl oz) chicken or fish stock

1 cup (250 ml/9 fl oz) reduced-fat or light coconut milk

500 g (1 lb 2 oz) raw prawns (shrimp), peeled and deveined

200 g (7 oz) firm tofu, cut into cubes

juice of 1 lime

½ cup mint leaves

2 cups (230 g/8 oz) bean shoots

1 Lebanese (short) cucumber, grated

4 small red chillies, finely chopped

SERVES 4

Place dried noodles (if using) in a large bowl and cover with boiling water for 3–5 minutes. Drain.

Heat oil in a large, high-sided non-stick frying pan over medium–high heat, then stir-fry lemongrass for 1–2 minutes, add laksa paste and stir until aromatic. Pour in stock and coconut milk and bring to the boil. Simmer for a couple of minutes to develop flavours. Add prawns and tofu and cook only until prawns are opaque. Add lime juice and remove from heat.

Divide noodles between serving bowls. Ladle laksa over noodles. Top with some mint and bean shoots and serve with a side dish of remaining mint, bean shoots, cucumber and chilli for personal taste.

DIETITIAN TIP
A healthy version of a great favourite.

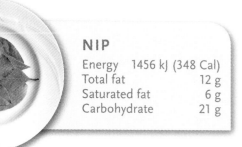

NIP
Energy   1456 kJ (348 Cal)
Total fat   12 g
Saturated fat   6 g
Carbohydrate   21 g

FRESH SILKEN TOFU WITH FRIED PEANUTS

CHEONG LIEW

1 × 250 g (9 oz) very fresh, whole silken tofu, either Japanese or Chinese, soaked in iced water until you're ready to serve

2 tbsp dark soy sauce

1 tbsp light soy sauce

2 tsp Chinese yellow rice wine

½ cup (125 ml/4 fl oz) peanut oil

80 g (2¾ oz) small peanuts

1 red Asian shallot, sliced

SERVES 6

Carefully drain water off tofu without damaging it and put in a shallow bowl. Add dark and light soy sauces and rice wine.

Heat oil in a large frying pan and fry peanuts until lightly golden, remove peanuts from oil and put on top of tofu.

Using same oil that cooked peanuts, add shallot and fry until golden. Pour over tofu and serve. Oil must be very hot before pouring over the tofu so soy sizzles. The eating quality is having hot crunchy peanuts with ice cold tofu, toasted soy sauce and very hot oil.

DIETITIAN TIP
It doesn't always have to be about the meat – a vegetarian choice all would enjoy.

NIP
Energy   1183 kJ (283 Cal)
Total fat   26 g
Saturated fat   4 g
Carbohydrate   3 g

PARMESAN CUSTARD WITH TRUFFLED ASPARAGUS AND SEMOLINA CRACKERS

BRENT SAVAGE

When making custard, the aim is to get it firm without the eggs splitting from the solids. However, by taking the custard to the point that it splits, then chilling and re-blending it, the texture is firmer and more solid. This fun recipe is a sophisticated play on a favourite kids' snack – cheese on a stick.

PARMESAN CUSTARD

300 g (10½ oz) parmesan cheese, grated

200 ml (7 fl oz) milk

200 ml (7 fl oz) water

8 eggs

TRUFFLED ASPARAGUS

100 g (3½ oz) fresh black truffles, thinly sliced

1 tbsp olive oil

1 garlic clove, peeled

1 bunch asparagus, thinly sliced into rounds

SEMOLINA CRACKERS

150 ml (5 fl oz) milk

25 g (1 oz) butter

1⅔ cups (250 g/9 oz) plain (all-purpose) flour

75 g (2½ oz) fine semolina

1 tsp sea salt

1 tsp baking powder

SERVES 6

NIP

Energy	2366 kJ (565 Cal)
Total fat	29 g
Saturated fat	15 g
Carbohydrate	42 g

For custard, combine parmesan, milk and water in a saucepan over low–medium heat. Cook, stirring, until parmesan melts into milk and water. Turn heat to low, whisk in eggs and continue whisking until mixture thickens and reaches 85°C (185°F). Chill mixture until it sets firm, then blend until smooth in a blender or food processor. Place in a piping bag.

For asparagus, blend truffles with oil and garlic to form a coarse paste. Marinate asparagus in truffle mixture for 1 hour before serving.

Preheat oven to 170°C (325°F/Gas 3). Line a baking tray with baking paper.

For crackers, in a saucepan, combine milk and butter and heat to 60°C (140°F). In a mixer, using a dough hook, combine all dry ingredients. While mixer is turning, gradually pour in milk and butter mixture. Continue to mix on slow speed until dough is smooth. Cover with plastic wrap and rest in fridge for 20 minutes. Using a pasta machine, roll dough out to lowest setting (about 1 mm/¹⁄₃₂ in thick). Cut into 3-cm (1¼-in) squares, place on a baking tray and put in the oven for 10 minutes. Remove from oven and cool on tray.

Pipe parmesan custard onto serving plates. Spoon truffled asparagus over top and stand crackers in parmesan custard.

DIETITIAN TIP
A recipe for a special-occasion meal.

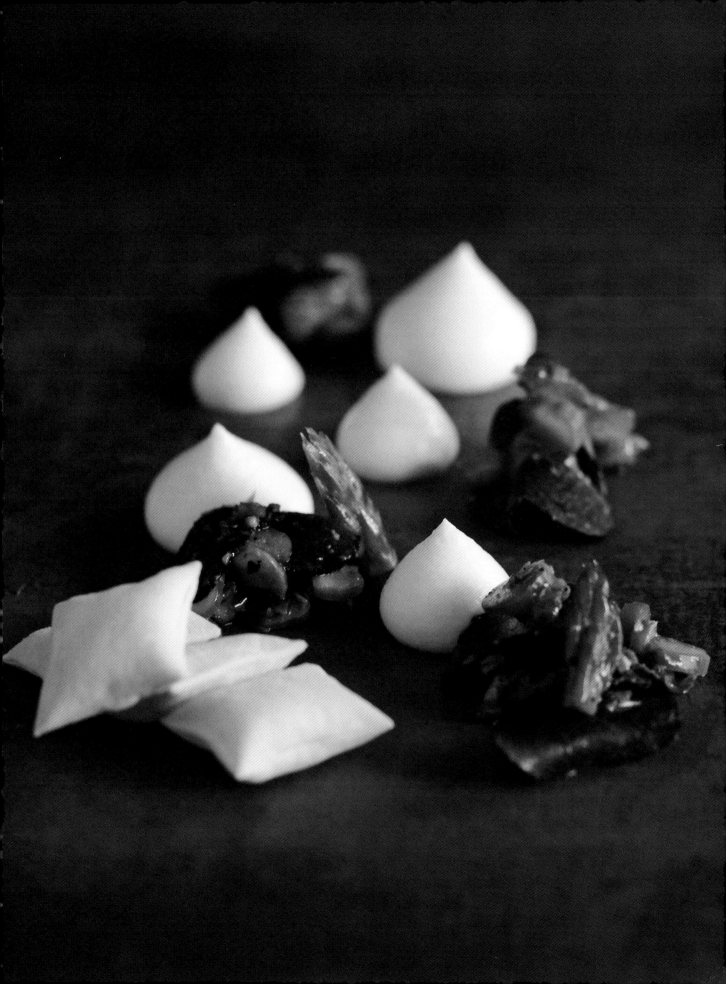

PRAWN TARTARE WITH STERLING CAVIAR AND SOY MIRIN DRESSING

GREG DOYLE

320 g (11¼ oz) raw tiger prawns (shrimp), peeled and deveined

2 tbsp extra virgin olive oil

2 tbsp snipped chives

12 baby golden mushrooms

12 baby garlic chives

12 red radish leaves

12 pea shoot tendrils

20 g (¾ oz) Sterling caviar

SOY MIRIN DRESSING

2½ tbsp soy sauce

200 ml (7 fl oz) mirin

2 thin slices ginger

juice of ½ lemon

SERVES 4

For soy mirin dressing, combine soy sauce, mirin and ginger in a small saucepan and bring just to the boil. Remove from heat and add lemon juice. Allow to cool and refrigerate in an airtight container until required.

Slice the prawns in half lengthways then dice them into 5-mm (¼-in) pieces.

Place diced prawns in a bowl with olive oil and chives. Divide prawn mixture into four equal amounts, place on serving plates and mould into a circular shape. Place mushrooms and herbs around prawn tartare and carefully pour on soy mirin dressing, making sure to avoid splashing tartare mixture. Finish by topping tartare with caviar.

This recipe is from *Pier* by Greg Doyle with Grant King and Katrina Kanetani (Murdoch Books, 2007).

DIETITIAN TIP
The carbohydrate here comes from the mirin.

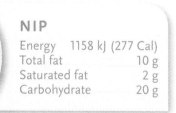

NIP
Energy	1158 kJ (277 Cal)
Total fat	10 g
Saturated fat	2 g
Carbohydrate	20 g

TUNA TARTARE WITH CRUSHED PEAS AND GOAT'S CURD

ANDREW McCONNELL

Raw fish and goat's curd — whoever thought! This combination, first brought to light by Tetsuya Wakuda, is a startling one. On their own, all three key ingredients – crushed peas, goat's curd and marinated tuna – have an individual intensity but together they form a harmonious dish. For a fresh entrée, team the pea salad with seared scallops.

½ garlic clove, peeled

1 anchovy fillet

1 tbsp light soy sauce

pinch of caster (superfine) sugar

2 tbsp olive oil

1 tsp balsamic vinegar

finely grated zest of ¼ lemon

250 g (9 oz) sashimi-grade tuna, trimmed and cut into 1.5-cm (⅝-in) cubes

1 cup (155 g/5½ oz) fresh shelled peas

3 tbsp extra virgin olive oil

1 tbsp lemon juice

1 French shallot, finely diced

20 mint leaves, shredded

sea salt and freshly ground white pepper

3 tbsp fresh goat's curd

8 pea shoot tendrils

SERVES 4

Use a mortar and pestle to crush garlic and anchovy, then transfer to a bowl. Whisk in soy sauce, sugar, olive oil, vinegar and lemon zest. Add tuna and leave to marinate in fridge for 15 minutes, stirring gently every so often.

Meanwhile, blanch peas in salted boiling water for 2 minutes, or until tender, and refresh in iced water. Using a mortar and pestle, gently crush peas to a very coarse-textured purée. Transfer to a bowl and add extra virgin olive oil, lemon juice, shallot and mint. Mix well, seasoning with salt and pepper to taste.

To serve, divide goat's curd evenly between four entrée plates and, with the back of a spoon, spread curd out to form a 5-cm (2-in) long rectangle. Arrange crushed peas over curd. Season tuna with a pinch of salt and, using a slotted spoon, remove tuna from marinade and carefully arrange over crushed peas. Dress plate with a few pea shoot tendrils.

DIETITIAN TIP
Goat's curd, a low-fat cheese, is best consumed soon after purchase.

NIP
Energy	1052 kJ (251 Cal)
Total fat	21 g
Saturated fat	4 g
Carbohydrate	4 g

GLOBE ARTICHOKES SIMMERED IN OLIVE OIL WITH GREMOLATA AND TOASTED CRUMBS

SEAN MORAN

A true artichoke aficionado, my Tuscan friend Sebastiano, who revels at being handed a whole thistle snapped straight off the bush, is the one who introduced me to this treat. The ceremony novel to me, I soon caught on as we dipped each leaf into a bowl of fruity olive oil and scraped the slightly sweet and nutty flesh from each leaf. I've since realised that growing your own is the key to this delicacy, ensuring the artichokes are 'squeaking' fresh. If you don't grow your own, try simmering bought artichokes in a dressing, and serve them loosely stuffed with herbs and toasted crumbs. Goat's cheese adds an interesting complexity, although someone like Sebastiano might consider it a bastardisation.

4 cups (1 litre/35 fl oz) extra virgin olive oil

6 garlic cloves, peeled

several oregano leaves, roughly chopped

several sage leaves, roughly chopped

several thyme sprigs

150 ml (5 fl oz) dry white wine

2 lemons

4–6 globe artichokes

sea salt and freshly ground black pepper

1 handful coarse fresh breadcrumbs

2 handfuls flat-leaf (Italian) parsley leaves

SERVES 4–6

Pour oil into a large lidded enamelled cast-iron saucepan into which artichokes will fit snugly. Coarsely smash 4 garlic cloves, then add to oil with oregano, sage, thyme and wine. Zest and juice 1 lemon and add to pan.

Trim about 3 cm (1¼ in) from top of each artichoke, then cut away (but keep) stalks so flower will sit flat. Discard a few darker outside leaves and tidy up any fibres with a sharp knife, then submerge in oil. Carefully peel each stalk to its paler centre, keeping it smooth and as round as possible. Add these to oil as well and season generously.

Bring pan to the boil over medium heat, then reduce to a steady simmer until stalks are just tender, about 25 minutes. Remove stalks with a slotted spoon and leave to cool. Return pan to heat and simmer until artichoke hearts are tender, about another 25 minutes. Remove with a slotted spoon and allow to cool. Keep cooking juices in pan – these will become the dressing later on.

Add a spoonful of oil from very top of artichoke pan (avoiding liquid at bottom) to a frying pan and heat over medium heat, then sauté breadcrumbs until deep golden. Drain on paper towel.

Meanwhile, make gremolata by removing zest from remaining lemon and mincing it with parsley and remaining garlic cloves.

When artichokes are cool enough to handle, carefully part centre leaves to reveal fibrous, furry 'choke'. Use a teaspoon to carefully scoop this out and discard. Open up flower and loosely stuff gremolata and breadcrumbs between leaves and in heart. Stir cooking juices well and check seasoning, then drizzle generously over artichoke hearts and stalks and serve.

DIETITIAN TIP

Although this recipe uses a large quantity of olive oil to cook the artichokes, the overall amount of oil will be around 1 tablespoon on each plate.

NIP
Based on 6 serves

Energy	988 kJ (236 Cal)
Total fat	19 g
Saturated fat	3 g
Carbohydrate	4 g

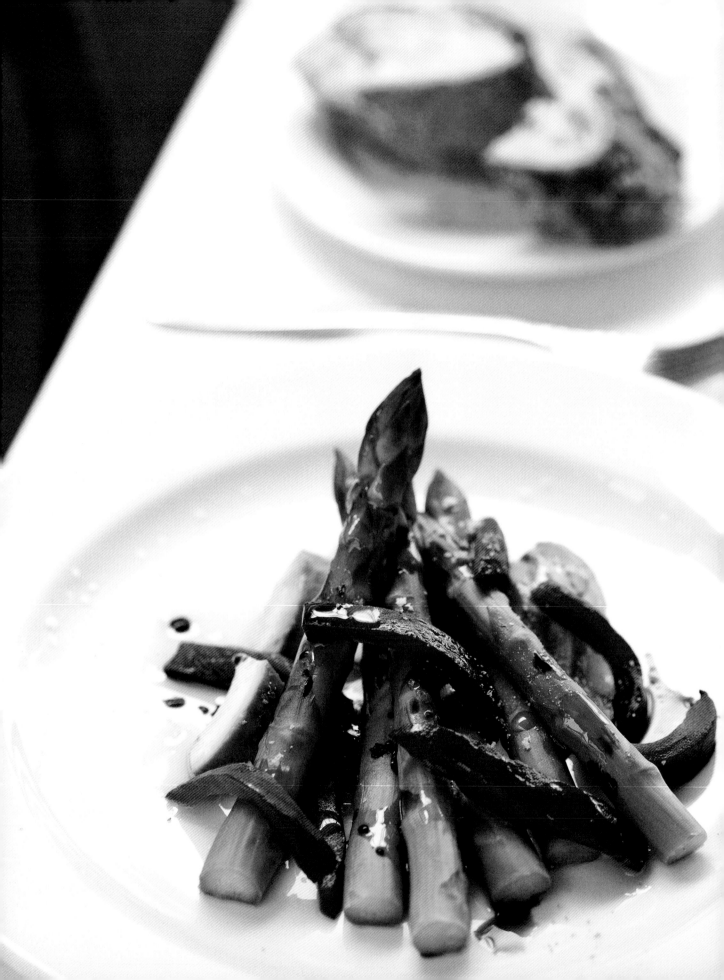

GRILLED RED CAPSICUM, ASPARAGUS AND AVOCADO – A SIMPLE SALAD

DAMIEN PIGNOLET

For those who believe that less is more, here is a pretty salad calling for the best raw ingredients at the market. Use equal proportions of each vegetable and allow enough to cater adequately for those about to enjoy this lovely dish.

2 red capsicums (peppers)

18 thick or 24 thin asparagus spears, trimmed

2 ripe avocados

best quality extra virgin olive oil, for drizzling

aged balsamic vinegar, for drizzling

sea salt and freshly ground white pepper

SERVES 6

Grill (broil) capsicum over an open gas flame or better still on a barbecue. Peel and cut them into 1-cm (½-in) strips, discarding inner membrane and seeds (never put grilled capsicums near water as this diminishes their flavour).

Blanch asparagus in a shallow pan of boiling water for 2–4 minutes, depending on thickness – they should emerge with some firmness. Refresh under cold running water and drain well, then turn out onto a clean tea towel to absorb any remaining water.

Cut avocados in half lengthways, then remove stones. Cut avocados into quarters and peel them, then lay on a chopping board. Cut avocado sections on the diagonal into 4–5 slices, then arrange on six entrée plates.

Place a bundle of asparagus around avocado and finish with capsicum. Splash with oil and a few drops of vinegar. Scatter with a little flaked salt and a few grinds of coarse white pepper. Serve at once.

This recipe is from *Salades* by Damien Pignolet (Penguin/Lantern, 2010).

DIETITIAN TIP
Drizzle on less oil and this recipe becomes very low energy.

NIP
Energy	939 kJ (224 Cal)
Total fat	22 g
Saturated fat	5 g
Carbohydrate	2 g

MARINATED SCAMPI WITH FRESH GOAT'S CURD AND JUNSAI

TETSUYA WAKUDA

250 g (9 oz) silken tofu

1 tbsp fresh goat's curd

sea salt and freshly ground pepper

1 tbsp cornflour (cornstarch)

6 scampi (allow 1½ scampi per person), peeled and deveined, shells reserved

½ tsp finely chopped French shallots

½ tsp walnut oil

½ tsp extra virgin olive oil, plus extra

½ tsp banyuls vinegar

pinch of chopped tarragon

20 g (¾ oz) salted frozen wakame, thawed, rinsed free of salt and cut into 1.5-cm (⅝-in) squares

finely snipped chives

16 pieces junsai (see note)

SCAMPI STOCK

shells from peeled scampi

100 g (3½ oz) diced carrot

100 g (3½ oz) diced onion

50 g (1¾ oz) diced celery

5 black peppercorns

2 bay leaves

2 tbsp thyme

2 tbsp tomato paste (concentrated purée)

SERVES 4

NIP

Energy	653 kJ (156 Cal)
Total fat	5 g
Saturated fat	1 g
Carbohydrate	8 g

For scampi stock, put first 7 ingredients into a large saucepan and just cover with water. Bring to a simmer, add tomato paste and simmer for 20 minutes. Strain, return to pan and reduce for 10–15 minutes till flavoursome but not bitter. Cool and reserve.

Bring silken tofu to room temperature. Pour off liquid and mix with goat's curd. Season well.

It is important that all ingredients are the same temperature before plating and serving.

For scampi essence, bring stock to a simmer. Thicken slightly with a slurry of cornflour and water mixed together. Remove from heat and set aside.

Cut scampi into six even pieces per tail. Just before serving, combine scampi, shallot, walnut oil, extra virgin olive oil, vinegar and tarragon in a bowl. Season with salt and mix gently together. Set aside.

In the centre of each serving bowl, arrange wakame in a thin layer. Gently spoon one-quarter of the tofu and goat's curd mixture onto wakame, making an even layer. Place 9 pieces of marinated scampi on top of tofu mixture and make sure layering is even and stable. Place a large pinch of chives in centre of scampi layer (to provide grip for the junsai). Arrange 4 pieces of junsai on top of scampi and dress with scampi essence, only 3–5 drops depending on strength. Drizzle on a little extra virgin olive oil.

NOTE: A preserved water lily with a gelatinous texture, junsai is available from Asian grocers.

DIETITIAN TIP
A very low fat and healthy entrée choice.

SCALLOPS WITH BLUE CHEESE POLENTA AND SHIITAKE MUSHROOMS

LUKE MANGAN

2 cups (500 ml/17 fl oz) water

pinch of sea salt

100 g (3½ oz) instant polenta (cornmeal)

2½ tbsp thin (pouring) cream

75 g (2½ oz) blue cheese, such as Stilton

50 g (1¾ oz) shiitake mushrooms, sliced

12 scallops, cleaned, with roe off

olive oil

1 handful watercress or baby rocket (arugula)

truffle oil, to drizzle (optional)

SERVES 4

To make polenta, bring water and salt to the boil. Pour in polenta in a gradual steady stream, stirring constantly. Cook over low heat for about 5 minutes. Stir in cream and crumble in blue cheese. Continue stirring until cheese is melted through.

Blanch mushrooms in salted boiling water for about 30 seconds. Drain.

Sear scallops in a little olive oil in a heavy-based frying pan over high heat, turning them once, until they just start to turn brown, about 2 minutes.

To serve, divide polenta among four serving plates and spread into a circle. Top polenta with a small pile of watercress or rocket and sprinkle with mushrooms. Arrange scallops around edge of polenta and drizzle with a little truffle oil, if using. Serve with a glass of chardonnay.

DIETITIAN TIP

By using small quantities of a strong-flavoured cheese such as Stilton, Luke Mangan has developed a reduced-fat entrée for us to enjoy.

NIP

Energy	978 kJ (234 Cal)
Total fat	11 g
Saturated fat	7 g
Carbohydrate	18 g

BRUSCHETTA OF RAW TREVALLY WITH SHISO, PRESERVED LEMON AND MISO RANCH DRESSING

DANIEL HONG

1 sourdough baguette

extra virgin olive oil, for drizzling

5 × 120 g (4¼ oz) sashimi-grade trevally fillets, skin removed, pin-boned

8 large purple shiso leaves, roughly sliced

½ bunch coriander (cilantro) leaves, roughly sliced

1 celery stalk, peeled and thinly sliced

1 preserved lemon, washed, skin finely chopped

1 bunch chives, finely snipped

3 tsp trout roe, to garnish

MISO RANCH DRESSING

100 g (3½ oz) sour cream

100 g (3½ oz) Japanese mayonnaise

2 tbsp full-cream milk

60 g (2¼ oz) white miso paste

2 tbsp lemon juice

¼ tsp sea salt

3 tsp onion powder

1 tsp garlic powder

SERVES 6

Make miso ranch dressing: whisk all ingredients together until smooth and well combined. Refrigerate until needed.

Preheat oven to 190°C (375°F/Gas 5).

To make croutons, slice baguette on an angle into 8 × 1-cm (3¼ × ½-in) lengths. Place them in a single layer on a baking tray lined with baking paper, drizzle with oil and place in oven for 7–8 minutes until golden and crisp but still a bit chewy in the centre.

Slice trevally into thin strips. Place in a bowl with shiso, coriander, celery, preserved lemon, chives and miso ranch dressing. Using a spoon, mix to combine well.

Place 1½–2 tablespoons trevally mixture on each crouton and garnish with a little trout roe.

DIETITIAN TIP
Low-fat milk, light sour cream and a low-fat mayonnaise would make the fat content of this dish much lower – but the flavour and texture will be rather different.

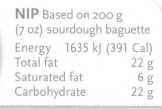

NIP Based on 200 g (7 oz) sourdough baguette

Energy	1635 kJ (391 Cal)
Total fat	22 g
Saturated fat	6 g
Carbohydrate	22 g

STEAMED DUCK, WINTER MELON AND SHIITAKE MUSHROOM SOUP

MARTIN BOETZ

60 g (2¼ oz) peeled garlic

30 g (1 oz) coriander (cilantro) roots, cleaned

60 g (2¼ oz) ginger, peeled

5 g (⅛ oz) white peppercorns, ground

100 ml (3½ fl oz) duck fat

100 ml (3½ fl oz) shaoxing rice wine

60 g (2¼ oz) rock candy, pounded

150 ml (5 fl oz) oyster sauce

100 ml (3½ fl oz) yellow bean soy sauce

6 cups (1.5 litres/52 fl oz) chicken stock

4 × 150 g (5½ oz) duck leg quarters, trimmed of excess fat

250 g (9 oz) small winter melon (dong gua), peeled and cut into spoon- and fork-sized pieces

1 preserved Thai lime

12 shiitake mushrooms, soaked, stems removed

GARNISH

50 g (1¾ oz) Asian celery, finely shredded

60 g (2¼ oz) ginger, cut into julienne

30 g (1 oz) garlic chives, snipped into 3-cm (1¼ -in) lengths

SERVES 4

Pound garlic, coriander root, ginger and ground peppercorns using a mortar and pestle until well combined and a paste-like consistency.

Place duck fat in a heavy-based saucepan and add paste. Fry paste over medium heat for 5 minutes until the ingredients are brown and caramelised, crisp and nutty. Deglaze with shaoxing rice wine. Add rock candy, oyster sauce and yellow bean soy sauce and cover with chicken stock. Bring to the boil and skim.

Remove from the heat.

Cut each duck leg through joint into 2 pieces.

In a bowl that will fit into a steamer, place the duck, winter melon, preserved lime and mushrooms. Pour on strained hot stock almost to top and cover with baking paper and foil. Place over a large saucepan or wok of simmering water, cover with lid and steam for 1¼ hours, topping up water level during cooking if necessary.

Take bowl out of steamer and check duck is cooked: meat should fall easily off bone and winter melon should be almost translucent. Check seasoning, adding more soy sauce if necessary. At this point you can let soup cool and reserve for later use.

Place soup in a large heavy-based saucepan. Gently simmer for 10 minutes until hot. Add garnish and simmer for a further 5 minutes. Portion into individual bowls and serve.

DIETITIAN TIP
Much of the carbohydrate in this recipe comes from the rock candy.

NIP

Energy	2064 kJ (493 Cal)
Total fat	22 g
Saturated fat	9 g
Carbohydrate	37 g

WINTER SALAD OF PRAWNS AND FENNEL

JEREMY STRODE

This salad was inspired by my brother's first trip to Australia. I've been here twenty years, so it was very exciting. He's a diabetic and an airline pilot, so takes good care of his diet and is particularly fond of seafood. Fresh prawns are amazing in winter but frozen ones are fine. Jane cooked her Corn, clam and Thai basil soup (page 42) for him on one of the rare occasions we weren't showing off Sydney's restaurants.

1 large fennel bulb, trimmed

1 tsp olive oil

sea salt and freshly ground white pepper

1 handful rocket (arugula) leaves

1 handful flat-leaf (Italian) parsley leaves

1 handful watercress sprigs

12 cooked medium prawns (shrimp), peeled and deveined

12 orange segments, membrane removed

DRESSING

juice of ½ orange

1 tbsp sherry vinegar

1 tsp fennel seeds, roasted and ground

½ garlic clove, crushed

large pinch of sea salt

½ tsp freshly ground white pepper

100 ml (3½ fl oz) extra virgin olive oil

SERVES 4

Preheat oven to 170°C (325°F/Gas 3).

Cut fennel in half lengthways. Cut one half into 8 even wedges, reserve other half. Place fennel wedges on a baking tray, drizzle with olive oil, season and place in oven. Roast for 8–10 minutes until golden brown and softened.

Divide fennel wedges between four serving bowls.

In another bowl, whisk together dressing ingredients.

Finely shave reserved fennel half on a mandoline and divide evenly between bowls containing roast fennel. Add even amounts of rocket, parsley, watercress, prawns and orange to each bowl. Dress each salad, toss and serve.

DIETITIAN TIP
Watch the quantity of dressing if you wish to keep your fat intake low.

NIP

Energy	1245 kJ (298 Cal)
Total fat	24 g
Saturated fat	4 g
Carbohydrate	6 g

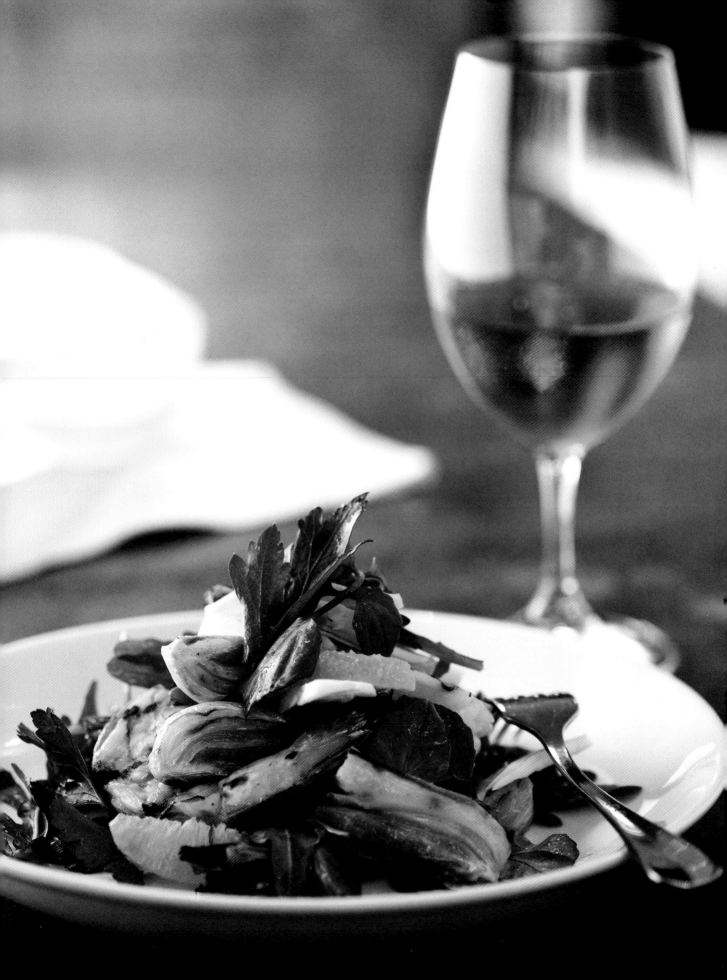

LAMB BRAINS WITH CELERIAC REMOULADE, BABY CAPERS AND WATERCRESS

JACOB BROWN

BRAINS

9 lamb brains

2 tbsp salt

½ onion, thinly sliced

2 thyme sprigs

1 bay leaf

½ celery stalk, thinly sliced

1 carrot, thinly sliced

8 cups (2 litres/70 fl oz) water

100 ml (3½ fl oz) white wine

½ cup (75 g/2½ oz) plain (all-purpose) flour, seasoned with a pinch of salt and freshly ground pepper

2 eggs, whisked

100 ml (3½ fl oz) vegetable oil

MAYONNAISE

2 egg yolks

2 tsp white wine vinegar

1 tsp dijon mustard

sea salt and freshly ground pepper

300 ml (10½ fl oz) vegetable oil

REMOULADE

½ celeriac, peeled and cut into fine strips

juice of 1 lemon

1 tbsp baby capers

1 tbsp dijon mustard

sea salt and freshly ground pepper

1 handful flat-leaf (Italian) parsley, chopped

GREMOLATA CRUMBS

1 cup (60 g/2¼ oz) panko (Japanese breadcrumbs)

3 tbsp finely chopped flat-leaf (Italian) parsley

1 garlic clove, finely chopped

grated zest of 1 lemon

TO SERVE

1 handful watercress

3 red radishes, thinly sliced

1 tbsp extra virgin olive oil

6 lemon wedges

SERVES 6

Cut brains in half to separate lobes, then soak them overnight in water with 1 tbsp salt to remove blood.

Place onion, thyme, bay leaf, celery, carrot and water in a suitable saucepan. Bring to the boil and simmer for 20 minutes to make a vegetable stock. Add white wine and simmer for 5 minutes longer. Add the remaining salt, then brains and turn off heat. Poach the brains for 5 minutes in this stock. Remove and drain in a colander. Place brains in fridge for 30 minutes to cool and firm.

While the brains are cooling, make mayonnaise, remoulade and gremolata crumbs.

To make mayonnaise, place all ingredients except oil in a food processor and blend until pale and creamy. With motor running, pour in enough oil, in a steady stream, until mayonnaise is thick. Only one-third of the mayonnaise will be used, the rest can be refrigerated in an airtight container for up to 10 days.

To make remoulade, place celeriac, lemon juice, capers, mustard, seasoning and parsley in a large bowl. Mix together well and stir in 4 tablespoons mayonnaise. Season to taste and place in fridge until ready to serve.

To make gremolata crumbs, mix all ingredients together.

Toss brains in seasoned flour, dip in whisked eggs, then coat in gremolata crumbs. Place crumbed brains in fridge to set for 1 hour.

Heat vegetable oil in a large heavy-based saucepan over medium–high heat. Add crumbed brains and fry until golden brown, then remove and drain on paper towel.

Place a little pile of remoulade in the centre of each serving plate, place cooked brains on top and finish with a salad of watercress and radish. Drizzle over extra virgin olive oil and place a lemon wedge on each plate.

DIETITIAN TIP
Like other types of offal, brains are high in saturated fat.

NIP
Energy	1950 kJ (466 Cal)
Total fat	39 g
Saturated fat	6 g
Carbohydrate	13 g

SCALLOPS WITH SAMPHIRE, SAFFRON AND SORREL

GEORGE BIRON

500 g (1 lb 2 oz) dry scallops (see notes) with coral attached

120 g (4¼ oz) marsh samphire (see notes)

4 French shallots, finely diced

100 ml (3½ fl oz) dry vermouth (Noilly Prat is good)

100 g (3½ oz) unsalted butter, cut into small pieces and chilled

pinch of pure ground saffron

100 g (3½ oz) French sorrel, shredded

1 tbsp extra virgin olive oil (a good workman-like Australian one)

sea salt and freshly ground pepper

squeeze of lemon juice

SERVES 6

Clean scallops by removing small intestinal tract and any adductor muscle that may be attached. Set aside.

Wash and trim the samphire, pat dry and set aside.

In a large saucepan over low heat, cook shallot slowly in vermouth until all liquid has evaporated. Add a little butter and the saffron and sorrel, and sauté gently until sorrel is soft and silken. Add samphire and heat through. Whisk in remaining butter. Set aside.

In a very hot, lightly oiled frying pan, sear scallops on both sides for about 30 seconds. Season and squeeze a little lemon juice on top. Taste and adjust seasoning.

To serve, divide saffron butter sauce between warmed plates and top with cooked scallops.

NOTES: Dry scallops are not soaked in water.

Samphire is available at good grocers. If you wish, you may substitute pickled or fresh seaweed for samphire.

DIETITIAN TIP
Half of the fat in this recipe is saturated fat – not the best choice for a regular meal if you have high cholesterol.

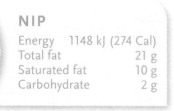

NIP
Energy   1148 kJ (274 Cal)
Total fat   21 g
Saturated fat   10 g
Carbohydrate   2 g

ABE'S FISH AND PRAWN CAKES

JENNICE KERSH AND RAYMOND KERSH

Our father Abe was a very proud Jew and a diabetic. He was also very liberal re religion, hence the forbidden shellfish as an ingredient. This was one of his favourite recipes.

Abe was an amazingly innovative cook who always thought that it was fine to break a cooking tradition if it improved the flavour and did not hurt anyone. These cakes are Dad's unique interpretation of the very traditional gefilte fish. They are delicious hot or cold.

500 g (1 lb 2 oz) ocean perch, bream or flathead fillets (the combination of fish must be one oily and the other a non-oily fish), chopped and skin removed

500 g (1 lb 2 oz) mullet fillets, chopped and skin removed

300 g (10½ oz) raw prawns (shrimp), peeled, deveined and chopped

2 tbsp chopped dill

2 tbsp chopped coriander (cilantro) leaves

1 large onion, finely chopped

1 large carrot, grated

1 long celery stalk, finely chopped

½ cup (60 g/2¼ oz) candlenuts, chopped

2 bird's eye chillies, finely chopped

2 eggs

sea salt and freshly ground pepper

1.3 litres (45¼ fl oz) fish stock, or water with a few slices of lemon added and seasoned with salt and pepper

1 cup (160 g/5¾ oz) rice flour

2 tbsp dry breadcrumbs

2 tbsp sesame oil

2 tbsp canola oil

200 g (7 oz) baby wild rocket (arugula)

extra virgin olive oil, to garnish

flesh of 6 finger limes, or 3 limes, quartered

SERVES 12 AS AN ENTRÉE (2 CAKES PER PERSON)

Mince fish in a food processor and place in a mixing bowl. Add prawns, dill and coriander, then onion, carrot, celery, candlenuts, chilli, eggs, salt and pepper. Mix until well combined.

Wet hands with water, then take a small handful of mixture and form into a patty or ball shape (for finger food, just make them half the size) and lightly poach in a saucepan of simmering fish stock or lemon water until cakes float to surface. A large pan usually fits about 6–8 cakes. Remove with a slotted spoon and place on paper towel.

While they are either still warm or at room temperature, dip fish and prawn cakes in rice flour and breadcrumbs. Heat sesame and canola oils in a large frying pan over medium heat and lightly shallow fry cakes on both sides.

These cakes are delicious hot or cold. Place them decoratively on a platter covered with rocket, drizzle with extra virgin olive oil and garnish with finger lime flesh, if available, or lime quarters.

DIETITIAN TIP
To minimise the absorption of fat into the cakes, make sure the oil is very hot before frying.

NIP
Energy   1174 kJ (281 Cal)
Total fat   15 g
Saturated fat   3 g
Carbohydrate   12 g

CORN, CLAM AND THAI BASIL SOUP

JANE STRODE

1 kg (2 lb 4 oz) clams (vongole), cleaned

1 tbsp vegetable oil

3 brown onions, sliced

6 garlic cloves, sliced

zest of 1 lime

100 ml (3½ fl oz) white wine

3 tbsp olive oil

6 coriander (cilantro) roots and stems, washed and chopped

ground white pepper

1 tsp sea salt

3 cups (600 g/1 lb 5 oz) fresh corn kernels

4 cups (1 litre/35 fl oz) chicken stock

fish sauce, to taste

3 tbsp thinly sliced Thai basil or coriander

SERVES 4

Soak clams in water for 1 hour to purge them of any grit. Drain and reserve.

Heat a large saucepan over medium heat and add the vegetable oil. Cook 1 onion and 2 garlic cloves until soft. Add clams, lime zest and wine and cover with a lid. Cook over high heat, stirring once or twice, for a few minutes, or until clams have opened. Pour clams into a colander, reserving cooking liquor. Remove clams from their shells and reserve. Discard shells and cooked onion mixture.

Heat olive oil in a large saucepan over medium heat, add remaining onion and garlic and cook for 5 minutes until they start to soften. Add coriander roots and stems, pepper and salt. Cook over medium heat until completely soft, about 20 minutes. Add corn, stock and reserved clam cooking liquor. Simmer for 20 minutes. Purée in a blender to a smooth consistency, then pass through a coarse strainer.

Season soup with fish sauce and serve warm with clams and basil or coriander sprinkled on top.

DIETITIAN TIP
Shellfish contains small quantities of polyunsaturated fat.

NIP

Energy	1753 kJ (419 Cal)
Total fat	22 g
Saturated fat	3 g
Carbohydrate	32 g

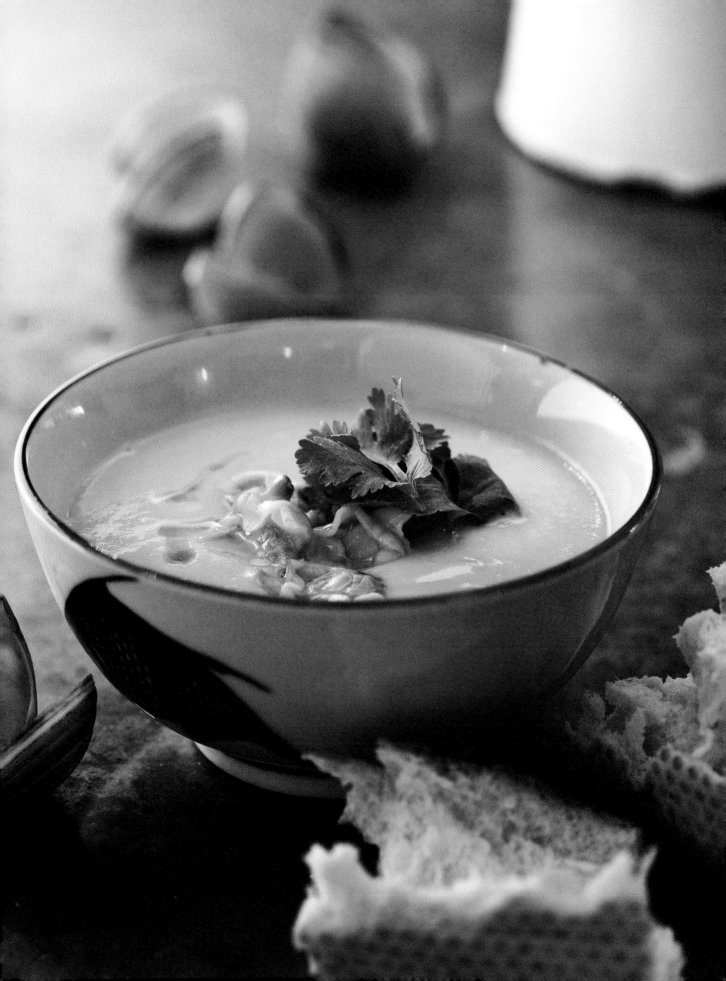

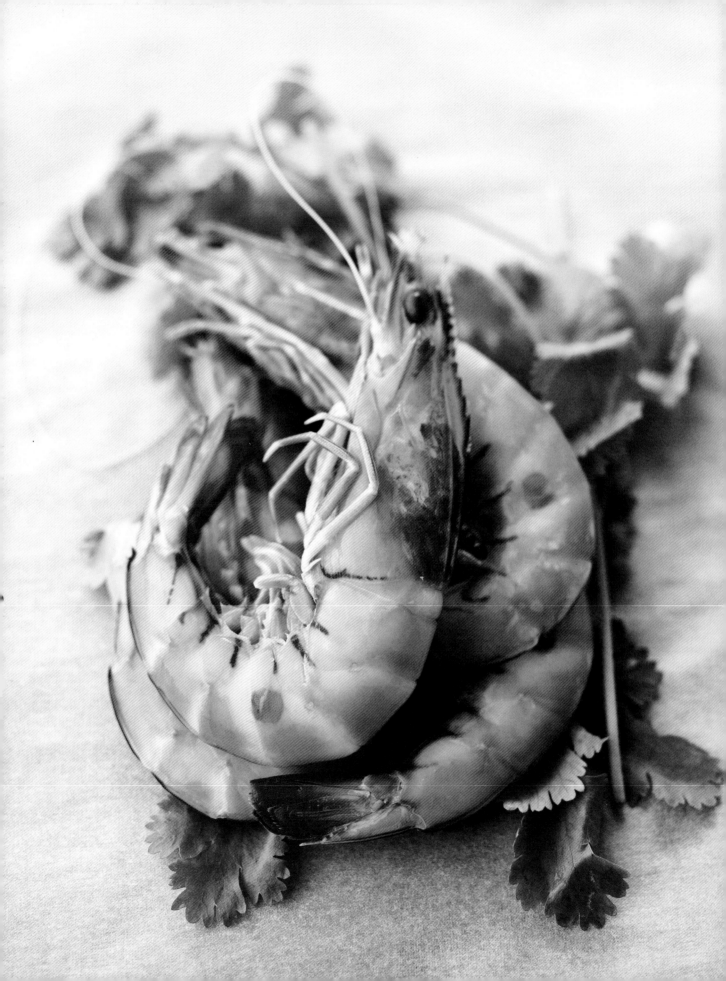

SEAFOOD

KINGFISH FILLETS WITH HERB CRUST AND FRESH TOMATO SAUCE

SERGE DANSEREAU

1 small handful flat-leaf (Italian) parsley, roughly chopped

1 small handful chervil, roughly chopped

100 g (3½ oz) dry breadcrumbs

1 garlic clove, finely chopped

finely grated zest of 1 lemon

⅓ cup (50 g/1¾ oz) parmesan cheese, freshly grated

125 g (4½ oz) butter, diced, at room temperature

4 × 180 g (6½ oz) boneless kingfish fillets (see note)

1 tbsp olive oil

fresh tomato sauce (see following recipe) or tomato passata (puréed tomatoes), warmed, to serve

SERVES 4

Put parsley and chervil in a food processor or blender and process until crushed and combined. Add breadcrumbs and blend until you have a smooth green paste. Add the garlic, lemon zest, parmesan and butter, and pulse until well incorporated. Scrape onto a large piece of baking paper, cover with another sheet of paper and roll out to make a thin dough, about 3 mm (⅛ in) thick. Refrigerate until needed.

Preheat oven to 200°C (400°F/Gas 6).

Wipe fish fillets with paper towel to remove any moisture. Take herb dough from fridge and sit it in the paper on a clean work surface. Peel off top layer of paper and place one piece of fish at a time onto dough. Use a sharp knife to cut dough and paper around contour of fish.

Heat oil in a large ovenproof frying pan over medium heat. Gently transfer fish to pan, paper side down. Cook for 3 minutes, or until you achieve some colour on crust. Turn over and cook for a few minutes in oven.

Remove from oven, peel off paper and serve immediately on warm plates with fresh tomato sauce as base. This dish goes well with a simple salad or steamed greens.

NOTE: Mulloway (jewfish), snapper or swordfish could also be used.

FRESH TOMATO SAUCE

2 garlic cloves, peeled

2 thyme sprigs

2 oregano sprigs

1 handful basil leaves

1 tbsp olive oil

sea salt and freshly ground pepper

8 roma (plum) tomatoes, halved

MAKES 2 CUPS (500 ML/17 FL OZ)

Preheat oven to 160°C (315°F/Gas 2–3).

On a baking tray, scatter over garlic, thyme, oregano and basil. Drizzle on olive oil and season with salt and pepper. Put tomatoes, cut side down, on top of herbs. Roast in oven for 30 minutes. Remove from oven and allow to cool slightly, then peel off skins. Reserve garlic and discard herbs.

Reduce oven temperature to 140°C (275°F/Gas 1), return tomatoes to baking tray and roast for 1 hour. Remove from oven and allow to cool slightly before using a hand-held blender to purée into a smooth sauce. Alternatively, you could do this in a food processor. Strain to remove seeds. Mash garlic and add to sauce. Pour sauce into a saucepan over low heat and cook for 30 minutes, or until it thickens. Adjust seasoning and reserve until ready to use.

Sauce can be stored in an airtight container in fridge for up to 4 days. Gently reheat sauce, and adjust seasoning with salt and pepper before using.

This recipe is from *French Kitchen* by Serge Dansereau (ABC Books, 2010).

DIETITIAN TIP
The carbohydrate content of this recipe comes from the breadcrumbs. For something a little different and higher in fibre, try wholemeal breadcrumbs.

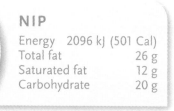

NIP

Energy	2096 kJ (501 Cal)
Total fat	26 g
Saturated fat	12 g
Carbohydrate	20 g

GRILLED SEAFOOD SPIEDINI WITH CABBAGE SALAD AND SALSA SALMORIGLIO

STEFANO MANFREDI

SPIEDINI

24 cherry tomatoes

8 raw king prawns (shrimp), peeled and deveined

8 scallops

2 garlic cloves, minced

1 large handful flat-leaf (Italian) parsley leaves, roughly chopped

4 tbsp oregano leaves, roughly chopped

juice of 1 lemon

3 tbsp extra virgin olive oil, plus 2 tbsp extra for frying

SAVOY CABBAGE SALAD

¼ savoy cabbage, tough outer leaves and core removed

½ cup (125 ml/4 fl oz) extra virgin olive oil

4 tbsp red wine vinegar

sea salt and freshly ground pepper

SERVES 4

For savoy cabbage salad, thinly slice cabbage and place in a bowl. Dress with olive oil and vinegar. Sprinkle with 2–3 good pinches of salt and toss well. Leave cabbage for 30–45 minutes, giving it a stir occasionally. When ready to serve, toss with a few turns of pepper.

For spiedini, on each of 8 skewers that have been soaked in water for 20 minutes thread a cherry tomato, a prawn, a cherry tomato, a scallop and finally a cherry tomato. Lay finished spiedini on a plate and refrigerate until you are ready to cook.

For salmoriglio, mix garlic, parsley, oregano, lemon juice and olive oil together in a bowl.

Just before cooking, remove skewers from fridge and brush with garlic and olive oil mixture.

Prepare a grill (broiler) or large frying pan by heating extra olive oil over medium heat. Cook spiedini on both sides until seafood is cooked through (about 90 seconds per side).

Serve spiedini with cabbage salad and some more of the salsa spooned on top.

DIETITIAN TIP
If you want to add carbohydrate, serve this with bread.

NIP

Energy	1746 kJ (417 Cal)
Total fat	37 g
Saturated fat	6 g
Carbohydrate	4 g

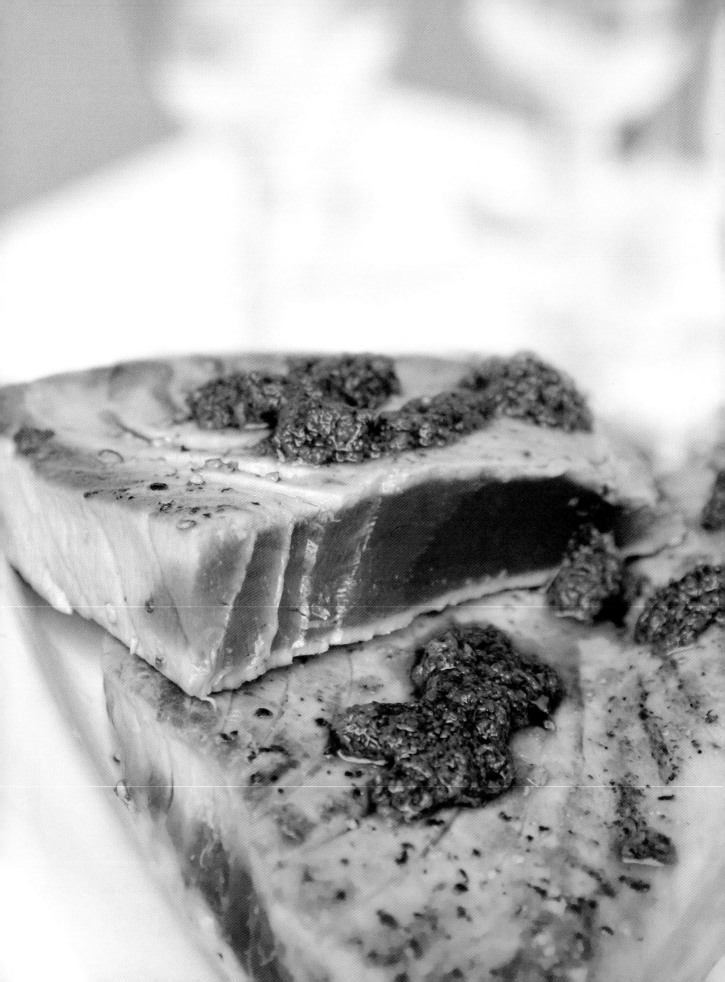

SEARED TUNA WITH SALSA VERDE

ROBERTA MUIR

*This vibrant green sauce will keep covered in the fridge for a week;
serve drizzled over any fish or meat, or as a dipping sauce for cold prawns (shrimp).*

4 × 200 g (7 oz) sashimi-grade tuna steaks
(see notes)

sea salt and freshly ground pepper

a little extra virgin olive oil

crusty bread, to serve

SALSA VERDE

2 large handfuls flat-leaf (Italian) parsley
leaves

4 garlic cloves, chopped

2 tbsp capers, rinsed

7 anchovy fillets (see notes)

½ cup (125 ml/4 fl oz) extra virgin olive oil

SERVES 4

To make salsa verde, combine all the
ingredients in a food processor or blender
and process until smooth.

Season fish well with salt and pepper.
Heat a frying pan over high heat until it is
very hot, add a little oil and cook fish on
one side for about 30 seconds, just until
well coloured, then turn and cook other
side for another 30 seconds, just long
enough to colour.

Remove fish from heat and leave to rest
for a couple of minutes before drizzling
with salsa verde and serving with crusty
bread.

This recipe is supplied by Roberta Muir from
FISHline, Sydney Fish Market's free consumer
advisory service.

NOTES: Remove the fish from the fridge about
20–30 minutes before you cook it, to allow it to come
to room temperature; this is particularly important if
it is being served rare in the centre.

Sashimi-grade fish is normally sold trimmed, but
if it is not, trim off any skin and dark muscle before
cooking. If available, use Ortiz brand anchovy fillets
as they have a much better flavour and are less salty;
1 small tin (47.5 g/1¾ oz) is the right amount.

Alternative species you could use are Atlantic salmon,
swordfish and yellowtail kingfish.

DIETITIAN TIP

Tuna contains some polyunsaturated fat so only
a little oil needs to be added during cooking.

NIP Based on a ⅓ of salsa
verde. Bread not included

Energy	1343 kJ (321 Cal)
Total fat	14 g
Saturated fat	2 g
Carbohydrate	0.4 g

CRISP-SKIN ROASTED SALMON WITH PUY LENTILS

BELINDA JEFFERY

If you have a special dinner coming up and you really want to impress, then this is the dish to do it. It's lovely – the salmon skin becomes wonderfully crisp and crunchy with beautiful tender flesh underneath. And what makes it terrific for entertaining is that it's so incredibly easy to make. The lentils can be prepared ahead so you only have to sear the salmon and pop it in the oven.

These lovely grey-green lentils are a French variety that are now being grown in Australia (here they're often called 'puy-style' lentils). They have a rich, earthy flavour and tend to keep their shape more than other lentils, so are perfect for using in salads.

1 cup (210 g/7½ fl oz) Puy lentils or tiny blue-green lentils

3 cups (750 ml/26 fl oz) cold water

4 salmon fillets, about 220 g (7¾ oz) each, skin on

sea salt, for rubbing

1½–2 tbsp extra virgin olive oil

½ red capsicum (pepper), roasted and finely chopped

1½ tbsp chopped flat-leaf (Italian) parsley

lemon wedges or slivers

DRESSING

1 tsp dijon mustard

½ cup (125 ml/4 fl oz) extra virgin olive oil

1–1½ tbsp red wine vinegar

sea salt

SERVES 4

Lentils can be very dusty and quite often hide little pebbles and bits of grit so it's important to give them a really, really good wash. To do this, put them in a big fine sieve and swish them around in lots of cold water in a bowl, changing water a few times. Then drain them and swish them around again under cold running water until water runs clear. It's a bit hard to see any little pebbles in lentils because of their dark colour but check as best you can.

Put lentils in a saucepan and cover with water. Bring to the boil, then reduce heat and simmer lentils for about 20 minutes, or until they're cooked but still have a nice little bit of 'chew' to them. Start checking lentils early on as cooking time can vary quite a lot, and they can rapidly go from perfect to overcooked.

While lentils are cooking, make dressing. To do this, spoon mustard into a large bowl and slowly whisk in oil. When it's incorporated, mix in vinegar and salt. Taste dressing and adjust flavours to suit you.

As soon as lentils are ready, tip them into a sieve or colander. Shake them really well to get rid of any excess water, then mix them into dressing. Leave them in a warm spot, stirring occasionally.

Preheat oven to 250°C (500°F/Gas 9).

Check salmon skin for any wayward scales. If there are some, just rub skin back and forth with the back of a knife, then rinse off scales. Pat fillets really, really dry and rub a little sea salt into skin.

Heat a heavy-based ovenproof frying pan large enough to hold salmon in one layer over high heat. When it's very hot, add olive oil and swirl it around to coat base. Lay salmon, skin side down, in pan and sear it for 2 minutes. Salmon skin shrinks as soon as it gets hot, which causes fillets to curl; to help prevent this, press down on top of fillets with back of a spatula to keep skin in contact with pan. As soon as 2 minutes is up, put pan in oven for 6–8 minutes, depending on thickness of salmon (a bit less if you like it rare, but you need to leave it long enough for skin to crisp). Once it's ready, carefully

remove pan from oven (watch out for handle as it will be red hot).

Stir capsicum and parsley into the lentil mixture.

To serve, spoon some lentils into middle of each of four warm plates. Sit a salmon fillet, skin side up, on top. Garnish with a fine sliver or wedge of lemon.

Fishy business: I hate to say it but there's one drawback with this dish and it's best to know about it before you start. The fishy smell from the salmon skin searing is pretty strong, so you do need good ventilation when you cook it. I usually have all the doors and windows open before I start cooking it, which can be a bit of a problem if it's arctic outside, but it sure beats eau-de-salmon for days!

DIETITIAN TIP
Lentils are a high-fibre accompaniment to this meal.

NIP
Energy   3630 kJ (865 Cal)
Total fat   58 g
Saturated fat   12 g
Carbohydrate   19 g

STEAMED MULLOWAY WITH SHELLFISH VINAIGRETTE

CHRISTOPHER WHITEHEAD

1 tsp olive oil

4 × 180 g (6½ oz) mulloway (jewfish) fillets, skin on

SAUCE

3 tbsp peanut oil

2 tbsp light soy sauce

1½ cups (375 ml/13 fl oz) fish stock

2 tsp sesame oil

VEGETABLES

3 tbsp peanut oil

100 g (3½ oz) oyster mushrooms, trimmed

50 g (1¾ oz) snow pea (mangetout) julienne

100 g (3½ oz) baby corn, halved

50 g (1¾ oz) French shallot batons

20 g (¾ oz) black cloud-ear fungus julienne

10 g (¼ oz) ginger julienne, blanched

1 bunch baby bok choy (pak choy), trimmed

coriander (cilantro) leaves

SHELLFISH VINAIGRETTE

75 ml (2¼ fl oz) shellfish broth

2 prawn (shrimp) heads

3 tsp verjuice

¼ tsp sea salt

sprinkle freshly ground white pepper

3 tbsp canola oil

3 tbsp olive oil

2 tsp tomato paste (concentrated purée)

½ tsp dijon mustard

SERVES 4

For sauce, whisk peanut oil, soy sauce, fish stock and sesame oil in a small bowl to combine.

For vegetables, heat peanut oil in a frying pan over medium–high heat, add vegetables and stir-fry for 2 minutes. Add 3 tablespoons sauce and simmer until vegetables are heated and sauce is reduced. Add coriander leaves.

For vinaigrette, combine broth with prawn heads. Simmer until reduced to 2½ tablespoons. Purée and pass through a fine sieve into a bowl. Whisk in verjuice, salt, pepper, canola and olive oils, tomato paste and mustard. Taste and adjust seasoning.

Pour a little olive oil on piece of plastic wrap. Place a fish fillet, skin side down, on the oil and wrap tightly. Repeat with remaining fillets. Steam fish for 8 minutes, covered, either in the top of a double boiler over a pan of boiling water or in a steamer basket in a wok. Unwrap the fish.

Place vegetables and sauce in centre of four pasta bowls. Drizzle over a little vinaigrette. Place a fish fillet on top of each and sprinkle with salt.

DIETITIAN TIP

White fish has a lower fat content than darker-fleshed fish such as tuna and salmon.

NIP Based on 1 tsp drizzle of shellfish vinaigrette per person

Energy	2279 kJ (545 Cal)
Total fat	39 g
Saturated fat	7 g
Carbohydrate	7 g

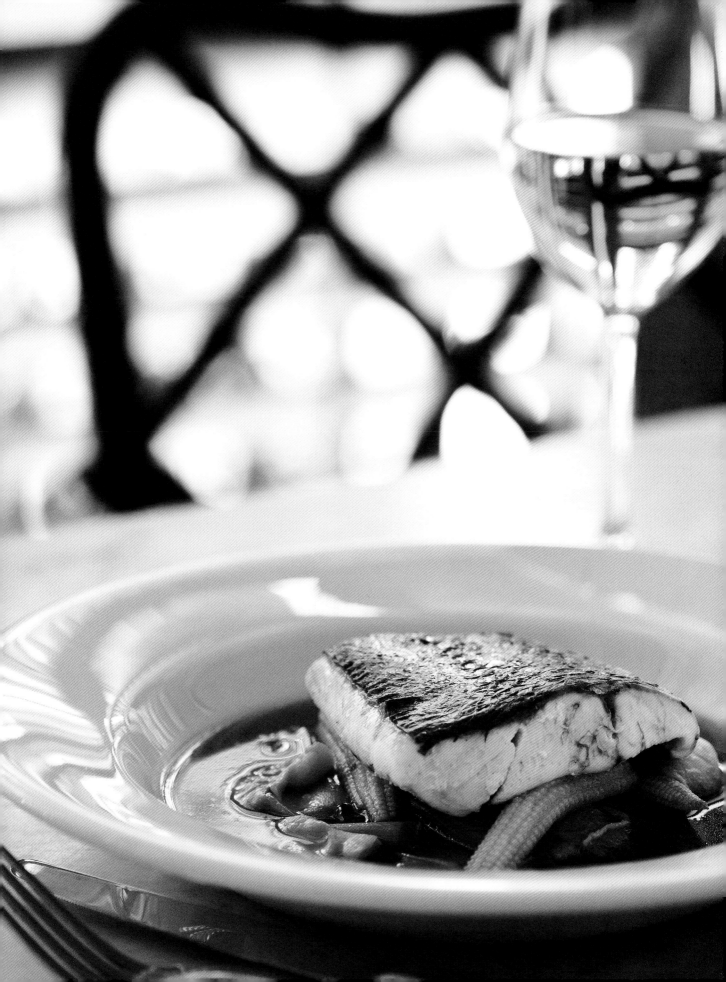

WHOLE SNAPPER BAKED IN A ROCK SALT CRUST, PERIWINKLES, SEA SCALLOPS, STONE POT RICE AND JAPANESE WHITE TURNIPS

PETER GILMORE

1 cup (210 g/7½ oz) sushi rice

2½ tbsp grapeseed oil

3 tbsp dried wakame

3.5 litres (122 fl oz) cold water

24 periwinkles

2 kg (4 lb 8 oz) rock salt

1 whole snapper, about 4 kg (9 lb), cleaned

32 small Japanese white turnips, green stalks trimmed, leaving 5 mm (¼ in) attached

16 scallops, cut in half horizontally

8 young samphire sprigs, broken into 2-cm (¾-in) long sections (see note, page 58)

100 g (3½ oz) mustard cress, tops trimmed

FISH HEAD AND SEAWEED GLAZE

3 snapper heads

100 ml (3½ fl oz) grapeseed oil

1 small knob young ginger, thinly sliced

½ bunch Asian spring onions (scallions), white part only, thinly sliced

300 ml (10½ fl oz) dry sake

8 cups (2 litres/70 fl oz) chicken stock

1 tsp dried wakame

40 g (1½ oz) sweet glutinous rice

white soy sauce, to taste

SERVES 8

To make fish head and seaweed glaze, cut snapper heads in half through middle with a sharp cleaver. You can ask your fishmonger to do this for you. In a very large saucepan, lightly brown snapper heads in grapeseed oil. Add ginger and spring onion and sauté for a further minute. Deglaze with sake and continue to cook until sake is almost evaporated. Add stock and wakame, simmer for 30 minutes over low heat, then add rice. Continue to simmer for 1 hour until reduced by half and slightly thickened. Strain stock through a fine sieve and discard solids. Return liquid to a clean saucepan and reduce until reasonably thick and you have about 2 cups (500 ml/17 fl oz) liquid remaining. Season to taste with white soy sauce and refrigerate until required.

To prepare sushi rice, wash three times in cold water. Place rice with an equal quantity of cold water in a rice cooker, or boil rice in a saucepan of water until cooked. When rice is cooked, remove half the rice, cover and leave at room temperature for no longer than 1 hour before serving. Add a couple of tablespoons of water to rice remaining in pan and cook for a further 10 minutes. The aim is to overcook this rice.

Take a tablespoonful of overcooked rice while it is still warm, place it between two sheets of baking paper and, using a large heavy rolling pin, squash and roll rice out very, very thinly, about 1 mm (1/32 in) thick. Leave rice between paper and, with a sharp pair of scissors, cut out a 20-cm (8-in) circle of rice and paper to fit a non-stick frying pan. Place rice and paper in pan and cook over low–medium heat for 1 minute. Turn rice and paper over, cook for a further 1 minute until rice is slightly firmer and drier. Peel away both sheets of paper. Add about 1 tablespoon grapeseed oil to same pan. Fry rice sheet for 1–2 minutes on each side until crispy and very lightly golden brown. Repeat this process so you have two 20-cm (8-in) crispy rice sheets.

Allow rice sheets to cool completely. Take one rice sheet and, with a sharp knife, finely chop sheet into small pieces. Tear the other sheet into 2-cm (¾-in) rough shards. Store shards and chopped rice in separate airtight containers until required.

Rehydrate wakame in 3 litres (105 fl oz) cold water for 1 hour. Remove from water, you should now have about 500 g (1 lb 2 oz) wakame. Tear seaweed into small pieces.

To prepare periwinkles, place them in a large bucket of iced water for about 30 minutes. This will send them into a coma, which relaxes meat when it's cooked and is a more humane way of killing them. Place periwinkles in a large saucepan of salted boiling water for 1 minute. Remove periwinkles from boiling water and place them straight back into iced water to stop

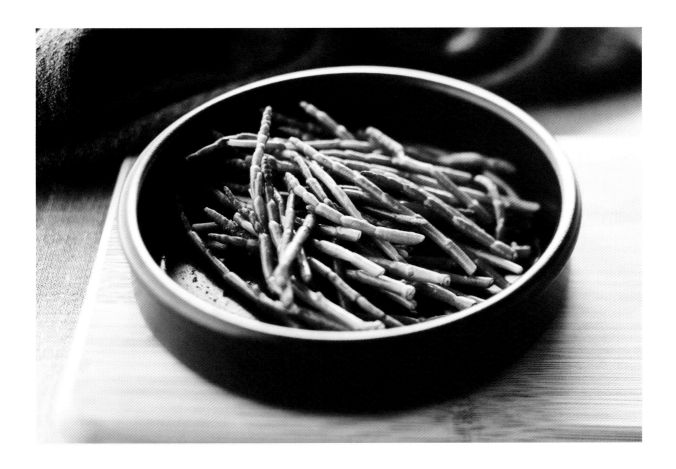

cooking process. With a thin metal skewer, hook and remove meat from shells. Discard intestines and cut meat in half vertically. Remove red mouth and place periwinkles in the fridge until required.

Preheat oven to 200°C (400°F/Gas 6).

Wet rock salt in 2 cups (500 ml/17 fl oz) cold water. You want salt wet. Do not add enough water to dissolve salt. Place half the rock salt on a baking tray and shape to form a mound roughly same size as snapper.

Cover snapper completely in wakame. Place snapper on bed of rock salt and top with remaining rock salt. Press salt around fish to completely encase. Bake in oven for 30 minutes. The only way to tell if the fish is ready is to crack open the salt a little. If it needs more cooking, return it to the oven. When it is cooked, remove fish from oven and allow to cool at room temperature for 10 minutes before breaking crust.

Lightly peel turnips and blanch in salted boiling water for 1 minute. Refresh in a bowl of iced water.

Break snapper crust with a blunt knife and peel away seaweed. Gently peel off skin and portion fish into 8 rectangles, using a sharp knife to cut flesh away from bone. Lift flesh off bone using a palette knife and cover with a clean tea towel. Keep warm. (Try to ensure you remove as many fine bones as possible when you are removing flesh.)

Divide glaze between two saucepans. In one pan, gently poach scallops and reheat periwinkles, baby turnips and samphire for 1 minute. In other pan, gently reheat reserved sushi rice for 1 minute and add mustard cress and finely chopped crispy rice.

Place 3 or 4 tablespoonfuls of hot rice mixture on each serving plate and add a portion of snapper. Ladle scallops, turnips, periwinkles and samphire around fish. Garnish with crispy rice shards and serve immediately.

NOTE: If you can't obtain samphire, use baby leeks instead.

DIETITIAN TIP
A great low-fat choice. With the rice included, this meal just needs some vegetables to make it complete.

NIP
Energy	2430 kJ (581 Cal)
Total fat	11 g
Saturated fat	3 g
Carbohydrate	35 g

WARM SQUID, LEEK AND CAPER SALAD

MAGGIE BEER

You can tell that I like squid — I cook it in so many different ways and want to encourage others to do the same. I cook the squid here in nut-brown butter, if it makes more sense to you, use extra virgin olive oil instead. The biggest tip I can give you is to only just cook the squid. However, if you've either cooked it a little too much or not quite enough, a generous squeeze of lemon juice will help to remedy both problems; it will either 'relax' the overcooked meat or 'cook' the underdone squid a little more.

4 pencil leeks, trimmed and cut into 12-cm (4½-in) lengths

extra virgin olive oil, for cooking

sea salt and freshly ground pepper

2 tbsp salted capers, rinsed

1 × 4 g (⅛ oz) packet squid ink

1 large lemon, zest removed with a potato peeler in wide strips, then juiced

3 tbsp verjuice

2 fresh bay leaves

2 tbsp marjoram leaves

3 tbsp olive oil

500 g (1 lb 2 oz) squid tubes, cleaned and cut into rings (or use cleaned baby squid, cut in half lengthways)

plain (all-purpose) flour, for dusting

100 g (3½ oz) unsalted butter, chopped

1 handful flat-leaf (Italian) parsley leaves

SERVES 4

Brush leeks with extra virgin olive oil and season with salt and pepper. Grill (broil) on a hot chargrill plate for about 5 minutes on all sides, or until caramelised and collapsed. Set aside.

Fry capers in 2 teaspoons extra virgin olive oil in a small frying pan over medium heat until crisp, then set aside.

Squeeze squid ink into a bowl and add a little lemon juice, then set aside.

Place lemon zest, verjuice and bay leaves in a saucepan and simmer over low heat for 5 minutes, or until lemon zest is translucent. Remove from heat, then add marjoram, olive oil and remaining lemon juice to taste. Set aside.

Toss squid in a plastic bag with flour seasoned with salt. Shake squid to remove excess flour.

Melt butter in a frying pan over high heat until nut-brown (or use a splash of olive oil if you prefer). Pan-fry squid in batches for about 1 minute on each side, or until golden; each batch needs to sizzle a little the moment it hits the pan.

Toss squid, leeks and parsley together and drizzle with squid ink mixture, then with verjuice mixture. Scatter on crisp capers and serve.

DIETITIAN TIP
If you wish to lower the percentage of saturated fat in this dish, use olive oil instead of butter to cook the squid.

NIP

Energy	1912 kJ (457 Cal)
Total fat	38 g
Saturated fat	16 g
Carbohydrate	6 g

MUD CRAB WITH CHAMPAGNE SAUCE

TONY BILSON

3 large mud crabs (4 kg/9 lb)

100 g (3½ oz) butter

6 French shallots, finely chopped

2 garlic cloves, crushed

3 thyme sprigs

1 bay leaf

freshly ground pepper

¼ tsp cayenne pepper

150 ml (5 fl oz) Champagne

150 ml (5 fl oz) fish stock

2½ tbsp cognac

100 ml (3½ fl oz) thin (pouring) cream

2 egg yolks

sea salt

3 tbsp chopped flat-leaf (Italian) parsley

SERVES 6

To prepare the mud crabs, chill them in iced water for 30 minutes. Lever the head shell from the body of each crab, then spoon any mustard and roe into a bowl and reserve.

Set aside the head shell. Remove the large claws and gently crack the shells with a hatchet. Cut the remainder of the crab into four pieces with two legs on each piece.

Melt butter in a very large saucepan and soften shallots and garlic over low heat. Add the mud crab, herbs and peppers and cook, turning the crab pieces, until shell begins to colour. Add Champagne and fish stock, cover with a tight-fitting lid, and cook over high heat for about 10–12 minutes until crab is cooked. Remove from heat. Strain liquor into a separate saucepan, and arrange the crab in a warm bowl. Bring the liquor to the boil, add cognac, turn down heat and simmer the sauce to remove the alcohol.

Meanwhile, beat crab mustard and any roe together with cream and egg yolks. Turn off the heat. Pass the egg mixture through a fine sieve into the cooking liquor. Mix thoroughly with a whisk and season with salt.

Pour sauce over mud crab and sprinkle with parsley. Have finger bowls on the table.

DIETITIAN TIP
Crab is a low-fat seafood choice.

NIP

Energy	1367 kJ (327 Cal)
Total fat	22 g
Saturated fat	13 g
Carbohydrate	1 g

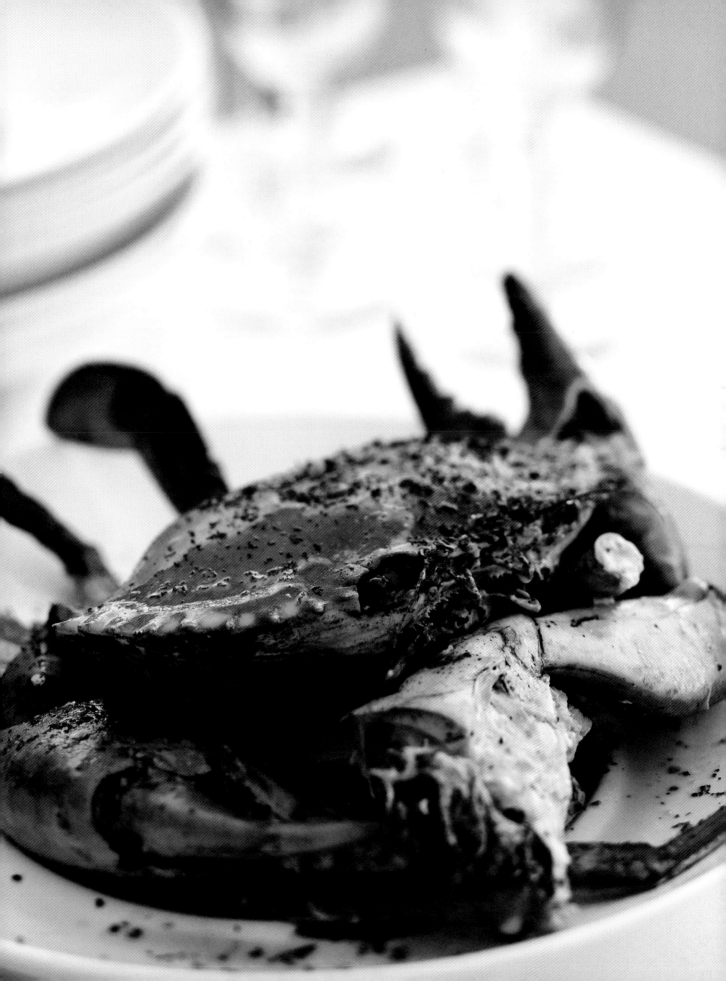

PAN-FRIED WHITING, SPICED CAULIFLOWER, WILD ROCKET, RAISINS AND FLAKED ALMONDS

PHILIP JOHNSON

350 g (12 oz) cauliflower, cut into florets

5 g (⅛ oz) unsalted butter

olive oil

⅓ cup (35 g/1¼ oz) flaked almonds, toasted

2 tbsp raisins

2 large handfuls wild rocket (arugula) leaves

juice of ½ lemon

extra virgin olive oil

plain (all-purpose) flour, for dusting

sea salt and freshly ground pepper

1 kg (2 lb 4 oz) whiting fillets, skin on, pin-boned (allow 3–4 fillets per person)

pinch of sumac

SPICE MIX

1 tsp coriander (cilantro) seeds

1 tsp cumin seeds

1 tsp fennel seeds

3 cardamom pods

⅓ tsp ground turmeric

CAULIFLOWER PURÉE

750 g (1 lb 10 oz) cauliflower, stems removed, chopped

1 bay leaf

full-cream milk, enough to cover

sea salt and freshly ground white pepper

50 g (1¾ oz) unsalted butter

⅓ cup (80 ml/2½ fl oz) thin (pouring) cream

SERVES 6

To make spice mix, toast coriander, cumin and fennel seeds with cardamom pods in a dry frying pan over medium heat until fragrant. Transfer seeds to a mortar (or use a spice grinder), remove seeds from cardamom pods, then discard the pods. Grind together, using a pestle, to make a fine powder. Combine with turmeric.

To make cauliflower purée, put cauliflower in a large saucepan with bay leaf and enough milk to just cover. Season lightly with salt and white pepper. Bring to the boil, then reduce heat and simmer until cauliflower is tender when tested with a knife. Strain cauliflower, reserving cooking milk. Gently heat butter and cream in a small saucepan. Place the cauliflower in a food processor and purée, gradually adding combined butter and cream. If purée is a little thick, add a little reserved cooking milk. Season with salt and white pepper. Set aside and keep warm.

Blanch cauliflower florets in salted boiling water for 1–2 minutes, then plunge into iced water to cool. Drain well.

Heat butter and a little olive oil in a non-stick frying pan over medium heat. Sauté cauliflower florets for 1–2 minutes. Once slightly coloured, add spice mix and toss in pan until florets are coated. Transfer to a bowl and toss gently with almonds, raisins and rocket. Dress with a squeeze of lemon juice and some extra virgin olive oil. Season to taste.

Season some flour with a little salt and pepper. Dust whiting fillets in flour, shaking to remove any excess. Heat a little olive oil on a barbecue flatplate or in a non-stick frying pan over medium heat. Cook the whiting for 1–2 minutes, skin side down, turn once, then quickly remove from heat.

To serve, spoon warm cauliflower purée into the centre of each serving plate and form into a circle. Place warm spiced cauliflower salad in centre and lay whiting fillets over top. Finish with a drizzle of extra virgin olive oil and a sprinkle of sumac.

NOTE: To serve as an entrée, reduce the quantity of whiting fillets to 500–600 g (1 lb 2 oz–1 lb 5 oz). This recipe is also delicious using scallops.

DIETITIAN TIP
You could make the cauliflower purée lower in fat by replacing the full-cream dairy foods with a low-fat variety but of course it will taste different!

NIP
Energy   2023 kJ (484 Cal)
Total fat   30 g
Saturated fat   11 g
Carbohydrate   10 g

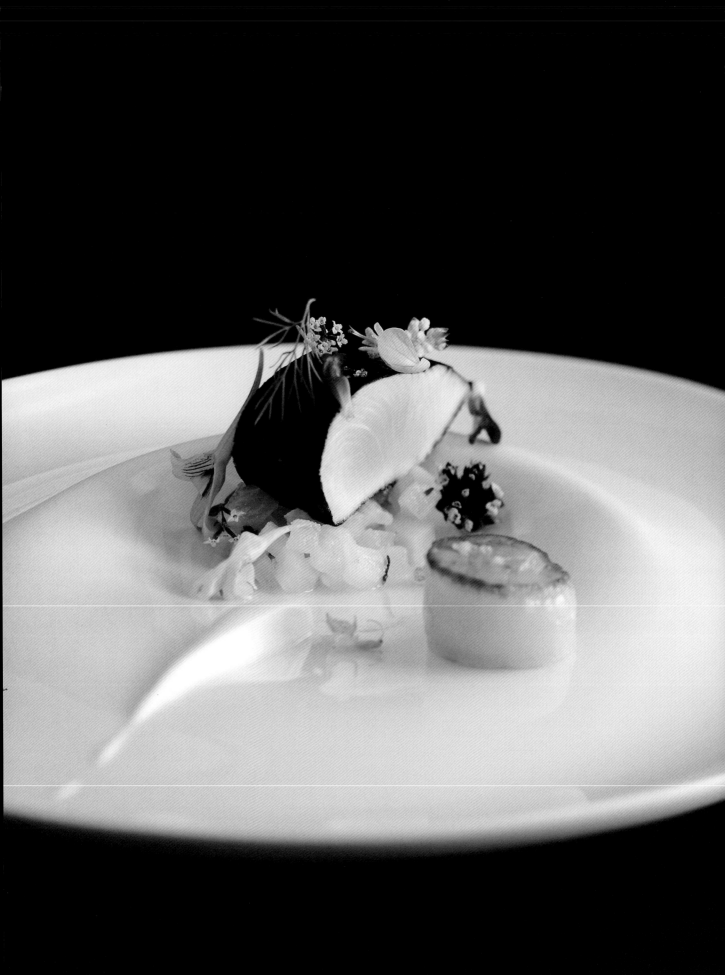

KINGFISH MARINATED IN SQUID INK WITH PERFUMED FRUITS AND COCONUT PURÉE

BRENT SAVAGE

6 scallops

edible flowers, to garnish

KINGFISH

40 g (1½ oz) squid ink

1 tbsp olive oil

pinch of sea salt

500 g (1 lb 2 oz) kingfish loin, cut into 6 equal portions

COCONUT PURÉE

1 cup (250 ml/9 fl oz) coconut cream

1 tsp agar-agar

PERFUMED FRUIT

1 semi-ripe mango, cut into 5-mm (¼-in) dice

1 nashi pear, cut into 5-mm (¼-in) dice

1 apple, cut into 5-mm (¼-in) dice

1 yellow peach, cut into 5-mm (¼-in) dice

dash of bergamot essence

3 tsp olive oil

SERVES 6

For kingfish, in a large bowl, whisk together squid ink, olive oil and salt. Add kingfish and rub fish pieces together. Individually wrap fish portions in plastic wrap or place in snap-lock bags and poach at 67°C (152°F) for 3 minutes. Carve ends off kingfish, then slice each portion in half lengthways. Set aside until ready to serve.

For coconut purée, mix 200 ml (7 fl oz) coconut cream and agar-agar together in a saucepan and bring to the boil, stirring constantly. Then simmer for 3 minutes and pour into a container to set. Place in fridge. When absolutely cold, place in blender and use remaining coconut cream to blend to a smooth purée. Pass through a fine sieve. Set aside.

For perfumed fruit, combine fruit in a bowl and dress with bergamot essence and olive oil. Set aside.

Sear scallops in a small frying pan over high heat for 1 minute, then turn and sear on other side for 20 seconds. Keep in a warm place until ready to serve.

Place perfumed fruit in the centre of each serving plate. Place a piece of kingfish next to fruit, and a second piece on other side of plate. Place scallops to one side. Spoon coconut purée next to kingfish, and garnish with edible flowers.

DIETITIAN TIP

The amount of carbohydrate in each serve is equivalent to one piece of fruit.

NIP

Energy	1048 kJ (250 Cal)
Total fat	13 g
Saturated fat	8 g
Carbohydrate	13 g

PAN-ROASTED FILLET OF BARRAMUNDI ON AVOCADO PEA MASH

DAVID PUGH

500 g (1 lb 2 oz) shelled fresh peas

2 tbsp olive oil

2 tbsp lemon juice

2 avocados, halved, peeled and lightly crushed with a fork

1 tbsp chopped flat-leaf (Italian) parsley

1 tsp chopped oregano

4 tbsp chopped mint

2 tbsp chopped coriander (cilantro) leaves

2 garlic cloves, finely diced

½ spring onion (scallion), finely sliced

1 long green chilli, finely sliced

sea salt and freshly ground pepper

6 × 160 g (5¾ oz) barramundi fillets, skin on, pin-boned

2 large handfuls salad leaves

6 lemon cheeks

SERVES 6

Cook peas in a saucepan of boiling water for 3 minutes and drain. Crush peas roughly with a fork. Mix peas, 1 tablespoon olive oil, crushed avocado, herbs, garlic, spring onion and green chilli to consistency of a chunky guacamole. Season to taste and keep warm.

Heat remaining olive oil in a frying pan over medium heat. Add barramundi, skin side down, and cook till crispy, 3–4 minutes, then turn to cook other side for another 3–4 minutes.

Spoon avocado and pea mash onto plates and garnish with salad leaves and lemon cheeks. For each serve, place a barramundi fillet on top of mash and serve.

DIETITIAN TIP

Pea guacamole – what a great idea. This is a higher fibre version of traditional guacamole.

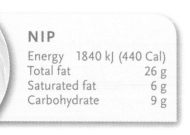

NIP

Energy	1840 kJ (440 Cal)
Total fat	26 g
Saturated fat	6 g
Carbohydrate	9 g

PAN-FRIED OCEAN TROUT WITH TOMATO, ROASTED RED ONION, OLIVES AND CONFIT GARLIC

LAUREN MURDOCH

2 red (Spanish) onions, cut into wedges

sea salt and freshly ground white pepper

vegetable oil, for roasting and pan-frying

1 tbsp lemon juice

30 garlic cloves, peeled

150 ml (5 fl oz) extra virgin olive oil

400 g (14 oz) grape or cherry tomatoes, halved

24 kalamata olives, pitted and roughly chopped

1 kg (2 lb 4 oz) ocean trout fillet, skin removed, trimmed and cut into 6 pieces

1 witlof (chicory/Belgian endive), sliced lengthways

1 large handful basil leaves, torn

SERVES 6

Preheat oven to 180°C (350°F/Gas 4).

Sprinkle onion with salt and pepper, toss in a little vegetable oil, place on a baking tray and roast for about 30 minutes until just golden. Remove from oven, toss onion in lemon juice and set aside.

Place garlic cloves in a small saucepan with olive oil. Heat over very low heat and cook for about 20 minutes until garlic is soft but not coloured. Allow to cool slightly.

Toss tomatoes with roasted onion, olives, garlic, most of the garlic cooking oil and some salt and pepper.

Season trout with salt and pepper.

Heat a frying pan over medium heat, then add a little vegetable oil and pan-fry trout for 2–3 minutes on each side, depending on thickness, until cooked to medium.

Divide witlof between serving plates. Add basil leaves to tomato mixture; divide most of this between plates. Place fish on top, then add remaining tomato mixture.

DIETITIAN TIP
Serve with a salad to improve the fibre content of this meal.

NIP
Energy   2097 kJ (501 Cal)
Total fat   36 g
Saturated fat   7 g
Carbohydrate   5 g

STEAMED SNAPPER FILLETS WITH GINGER AND SPRING ONIONS

KYLIE KWONG

4 × 100 g (3½ oz) snapper fillets

⅓ cup (80 ml/2½ fl oz) water

2 tbsp shaoxing rice wine or dry sherry

2 tbsp ginger julienne

1 Chinese cabbage (wong bok) leaf

½ tsp white sugar

2 tbsp tamari

¼ tsp sesame oil

½ cup (30 g/1 oz) spring onion (scallion) julienne

1½ tbsp peanut oil

1 small handful coriander (cilantro) leaves

pinch of ground white pepper

SERVES 4 AS PART OF A BANQUET

Place fish in a shallow heatproof bowl that will fit inside a steamer basket. Pour water and wine or sherry over fish, then sprinkle with half the ginger. Place bowl inside steamer and position over a large saucepan or wok of boiling water, and steam, covered, for 5–6 minutes.

Cut Chinese cabbage leaf into four squares and slip inside steamer. Cover and steam for a further 2–3 minutes, or until cabbage has warmed through and fish is just cooked. The fish should be white; if it is still translucent, cook for another minute or so.

Remove cabbage from steamer and arrange on a serving plate. Using a spatula, carefully remove fish from steamer and place on top of hot cabbage. Pour any liquid left in the bowl over fish, sprinkle with sugar and drizzle with combined tamari and sesame oil, then sprinkle with remaining ginger and half the spring onion. Heat peanut oil in a small frying pan until moderately hot, then carefully pour over fish. Sprinkle fish with remaining spring onion, coriander and white pepper, and serve immediately.

DIETITIAN TIP
Steaming is a great option for keeping the energy content of a meal low – no need to add any fat.

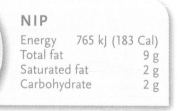

NIP

Energy	765 kJ (183 Cal)
Total fat	9 g
Saturated fat	2 g
Carbohydrate	2 g

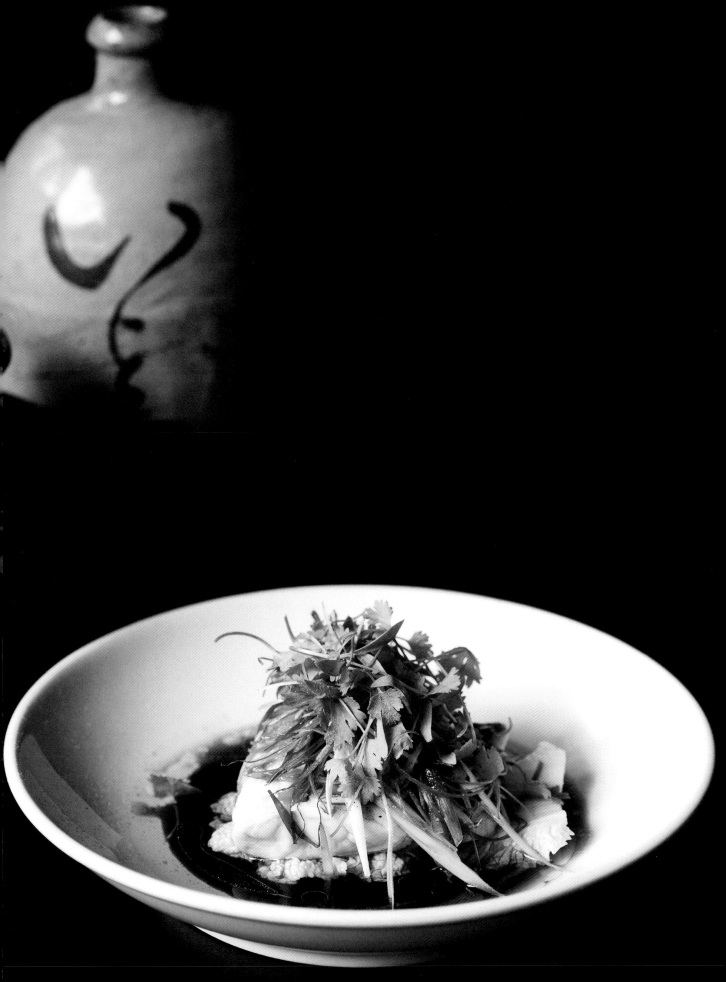

PAN-FRIED OCEAN TROUT, ASPARAGUS, FENNEL, FETA AND GREEN OLIVES

DAMIAN HEADS

1 bunch asparagus, stems trimmed

2 baby fennel bulbs, quartered

few strips orange zest

2 thyme sprigs

1 cup (250 ml/9 fl oz) extra virgin olive oil

vegetable oil, for frying

4 × 170 g (6 oz) ocean trout portions, skin on (see note)

sea salt and freshly ground pepper

GARNISH

120 g (4¼ oz) Persian feta, crumbled

¼ cup (45 g/1½ oz) green Sicilian olives, flesh cut off

¼ cup (40 g/1½ oz) thinly sliced red (Spanish) onion

1 small handful flat-leaf (Italian) parsley leaves

3 tbsp dill sprigs

2½ tbsp good-quality balsamic vinegar

SERVES 4

Blanch asparagus in salted boiling water for 2 minutes. Refresh in an ice-water bath. Cut asparagus at an angle into 2-cm (¾-in) batons.

Place fennel in a small saucepan with orange zest and thyme, then add enough olive oil to cover fennel. Allow it to cook over low heat for 40 minutes until a knife tip is easily inserted into fennel. Cut fennel into smaller pieces, reserve oil.

Place some asparagus and fennel on each main course plate, than arrange garnish. In order, arrange feta, olive cheeks, red onion, parsley leaves and dill sprigs.

Make a dressing with 2½ tablespoons reserved confit oil and balsamic vinegar.

To cook trout, heat a non-stick frying pan or barbecue plate over medium heat until hot. Add some vegetable oil and watch as it starts to shimmer – if it smokes, it is too hot. Season trout with salt and pepper. Place trout portions, skin side down, in hot oil and be sure to splash oil away from you. Cook fish on a gentle sizzle until it is visibly cooked halfway up side. Flip fish over, cook for 1 minute, then turn off heat. Allow fish to sit for a minute. Take it off when you are happy it is cooked the way you like it.

Spoon some dressing over and around garnish on plates, then place a piece of trout on top of each, skin side up.

NOTE: If the shop doesn't sell portions, use 800 g (1 lb 12 oz) trout fillet cut into 4 portions.

DIETITIAN TIP
As this recipe is higher in fat than some of the others, try keeping it for special occasions.

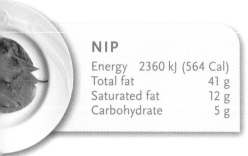

NIP

Energy	2360 kJ (564 Cal)
Total fat	41 g
Saturated fat	12 g
Carbohydrate	5 g

PAN-ROASTED MULLOWAY, BABY BEETROOT, FRIED CAVOLO NERO, PANCETTA, SAFFRON BANYULS

GREG DOYLE

80 g (2¾ oz) butter

12 baby golden beetroot and 20 baby red beetroot (beets), cooked (125 g/4½ oz per person)

20 cavolo nero leaves, stems removed and leaves shredded

150 g (5½ oz) pancetta, cut into 8-mm (⅜-in) dice

150 g (5½ oz) cooked Puy lentils or tiny blue-green lentils

50 g (1¾ oz) clarified butter

4 × 170 g (6 oz) portions mulloway (jewfish) fillets, skin on, pin-boned

50 g (1¾ oz) plain (all-purpose) flour, for dusting

SAUCE

pinch of saffron threads

150 ml (5 fl oz) banyuls vinegar

25 g (1 oz) butter, cut into pieces

SERVES 4

Preheat oven to 200°C (400°F/Gas 6).

Place two large saucepans on stove and add 40 g (1½ oz) butter to each. Add beetroot to one and cavolo nero to the other and lightly sauté each for 2–3 minutes until warm. In another saucepan, sauté pancetta until it is evenly brown, then add the Puy lentils.

Melt clarified butter in a large oven-proof frying pan over high heat. Dust skin side of fish with flour, then pat it to make sure any excess flour has been removed. Place a piece of baking paper on the flesh side of the fish. Place fish, skin side down, in hot pan, place a heavy-based pan on top of fish and cook for about 3 minutes. Then transfer pan, with other pan on top, to oven for about 2 minutes. Remove pan from oven and remove paper. Turn fish over, sear flesh side for 1 minute and then remove fish from pan. Keep warm while plating.

Meanwhile, make sauce by placing saffron and vinegar in a small saucepan over high heat. Reduce until a syrupy consistency forms. Whisk in butter pieces all at once to form a rich sauce.

To serve, first drag some sauce across each plate, then scatter beetroot and cavolo nero over plate. Make sure a line of lentils is added and then add fish last.

DIETITIAN TIP
The lentils add protein, fibre and carbohydrate to this recipe.

NIP

Energy	2165 kJ (517 Cal)
Total fat	28 g
Saturated fat	13 g
Carbohydrate	14 g

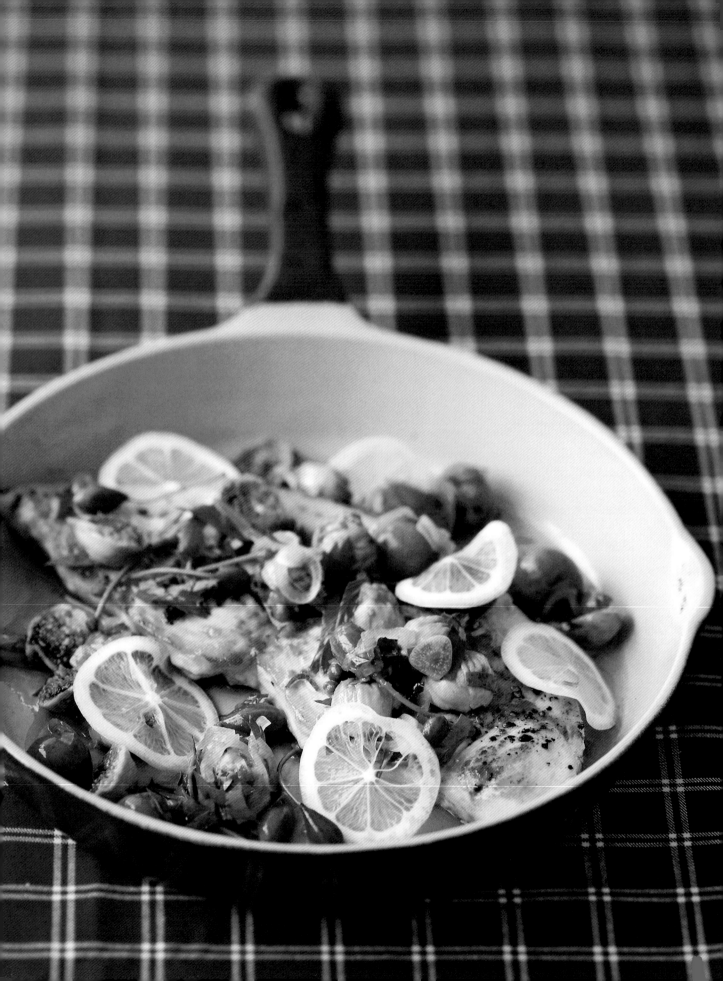

SWORDFISH WITH IRANIAN FIGS AND GREEN OLIVES

GARY MEHIGAN

*While I love all sorts of olives, I have a soft spot for the big green Sicilian ones,
which I have used here as they go brilliantly with the dried figs and a nice piece of swordfish.*

95 g (3¼ oz) dried Iranian figs

boiling water

⅓ cup (80 ml/2½ fl oz) extra virgin olive oil

1 French shallot, thinly sliced

½ garlic clove, sliced

1 cup (250 ml/9 fl oz) dry white wine

⅓ cup (60 g/2½ oz) green Sicilian olives

80 g (2¾ oz) small caperberries

sea salt and freshly ground pepper

1 large handful flat-leaf (Italian) parsley
leaves, coarsely chopped

2 tbsp olive oil

4 × 120 g (4¼ oz) swordfish steaks

1 lemon, very thinly sliced

fig vino cotto, for drizzling

SERVES 4

Place figs in small bowl and cover
with boiling water. Leave to stand for
10 minutes, then drain, discarding water.
Pat figs dry with paper towel, then cut
into quarters and set aside.

Heat a small saucepan over medium
heat, add 1 tablespoon extra virgin olive
oil. Cook shallot and garlic for 2 minutes,
stirring regularly; do not allow them to
colour. Add wine and figs, then increase
heat to high and reduce wine by three-
quarters. Remove from heat and add

olives, caperberries and remaining extra virgin
olive oil, then stir to mix. Leave to cool for
5 minutes. Season to taste with salt and a twist
or two of pepper. Add parsley, stir and set aside.

Heat a heavy-based non-stick or enamelled
cast-iron frying pan over high heat and add olive
oil. Season swordfish steaks with salt and pepper,
then pan-fry for 2–3 minutes (depending on their
thickness) on each side, or until tinged a light-
golden brown; they are best cooked medium-
rare. Remove from pan and rest for 2 minutes.

Place swordfish steaks on serving plates, then
spoon over fig and olive mixture. Divide lemon
among pieces of fish. Drizzle with a little fig vin
cotto and serve immediately.

This recipe is from *Your Place or Mine?* by
Gary Mehigan and George Calombaris
(Penguin/Lantern, 2010).

DIETITIAN TIP
The carbohydrate content of each serve
is equivalent to two slices of bread.

NIP
Energy   2005 kJ (479 Cal)
Total fat   33 g
Saturated fat   7 g
Carbohydrate   33 g

BLUE EYE FILLET BAKED IN LETTUCE LEAVES WITH BABY CLAMS, ZUCCHINI FLOWERS AND BOURRIDE SAUCE

JACOB BROWN

30 baby clams (vongole), cleaned

2½ tbsp white wine

6 × 200 g (7 oz) blue eye fillets

6 large iceberg lettuce leaves, blanched and refreshed in iced water

100 g (3½ oz) butter, melted

12 zucchini (courgette) flowers

3 tbsp olive oil

AIOLI

4 garlic cloves, finely chopped

juice of 1 lemon

2 egg yolks

1 cup (250 ml/9 fl oz) olive oil

½ tsp each sea salt and freshly ground pepper

BOURRIDE SAUCE

2 French shallots, sliced

1 fennel bulb, thinly sliced

2½ tbsp olive oil

2 garlic cloves, sliced

½ tsp coriander (cilantro) seeds, roasted

½ tsp fennel seeds, roasted

½ tsp black peppercorns

4 thyme sprigs

2 rosemary sprigs

2 bay leaves

2½ tbsp vermouth

75 ml (2¼ fl oz) white wine

200 ml (7 fl oz) fish stock

SERVES 6

Place clams in a large saucepan with white wine, cover and steam over high heat until clams open. Remove clams from pan and set aside.

For aioli, combine garlic, lemon juice and egg yolks in a blender. With motor running, slowly pour in olive oil until a thick, creamy sauce forms. Season with salt and pepper.

For bourride sauce, sauté the shallot and fennel in olive oil in a saucepan over medium heat until soft. Add the garlic and cook for 1 minute. Add spices and herbs and cook for 2 minutes to infuse flavours. Add vermouth and white wine, then reduce quickly until it reaches a syrup-like consistency. Add the fish stock and reduce for another 10 minutes. Season with salt and pepper. Then whisk in 3 tablespoons aioli and add clams.

Preheat oven to 180°C (350°F/Gas 4).

Wrap fish fillets in lettuce leaves. Brush with melted butter and bake in oven for 12–14 minutes, depending on thickness.

Sauté zucchini flowers in olive oil in a large frying pan over medium–high heat. Cook in batches for approximately 2 minutes on each side until golden brown.

Cut each wrapped fish fillet in half and place in a serving bowl, finish with clams, bourride sauce and sautéed zucchini flowers.

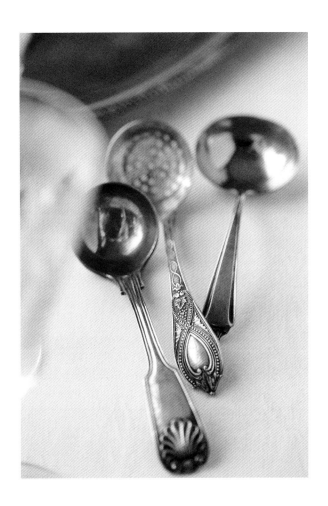

DIETITIAN TIP

If you want to reduce the fat and energy content of this dish, consider being careful with the bourride sauce and the aioli.

NIP
Energy	2555 kJ (611 Cal)
Total fat	44 g
Saturated fat	10 g
Carbohydrate	4 g

STEAMED BASS GROUPER WITH A TURMERIC CHICKEN BROTH

CHUI LEE LUK

I'd recommend using bass grouper in combination with other seafood such as clams (vongole), prawns (shrimp), crabs or even scallops to make the dish a substantial meal. I'd also add vegetables such as spring onion (scallion) batons, lightly stir-fried blanched zucchini (courgette) or steamed green beans.

4 × 100 g (3½ oz) bass grouper fillets

sea salt and freshly ground white pepper

TURMERIC CHICKEN BROTH

5 French shallots, roughly chopped

4 large garlic cloves, roughly chopped

1 × 5-cm (2-in) knob young ginger, roughly chopped

1 × 2-cm (¾-in) knob fresh turmeric, roughly chopped

finely grated zest of 1 kaffir lime

1 tsp white peppercorns

1½ tsp coriander (cilantro) seeds

½ tsp cumin seeds

2½ tbsp peanut or other neutral-flavoured oil

splash of brandy

10 chicken wings, chopped and roasted to light golden

1 lemongrass stem, white part only, bruised and tied in a knot

4 kaffir lime leaves

sea salt

SERVES 4

NIP

Energy	999 kJ (239 Cal)
Total fat	16 g
Saturated fat	3 g
Carbohydrate	1 g

For turmeric chicken broth, process shallot, garlic, ginger, turmeric and kaffir lime zest to a fine paste in a food processor. Roast spices until fragrant. Grind to a fine powder using a mortar and pestle or in a coffee grinder. Add to shallot paste. Place a heavy-based saucepan over medium heat, add oil, then spice paste. Cook paste until oil separates and comes to surface. Pour in brandy and cook until volatile alcoholic smell is dispelled. Add chicken wings, lemongrass and kaffir lime leaves, and cover with water. Add salt, bring to the boil and simmer for about 30 minutes. Let cool slightly, strain and discard solids.

Meanwhile, season fish fillets with salt and pepper, then place in a shallow heatproof bowl that will fit inside a steamer basket and pour some chicken broth over fish. Place bowl in steamer and transfer to a large saucepan or wok of simmering water, cover and steam until just done, about 10 minutes.

Transfer the cooked fish to serving bowls. Pour warmed broth over cooked fillets of fish, about 50 ml (1¾ fl oz) per person, and serve immediately.

DIETITIAN TIP

I agree with Chui that adding vegetables would be a great addition to this recipe.

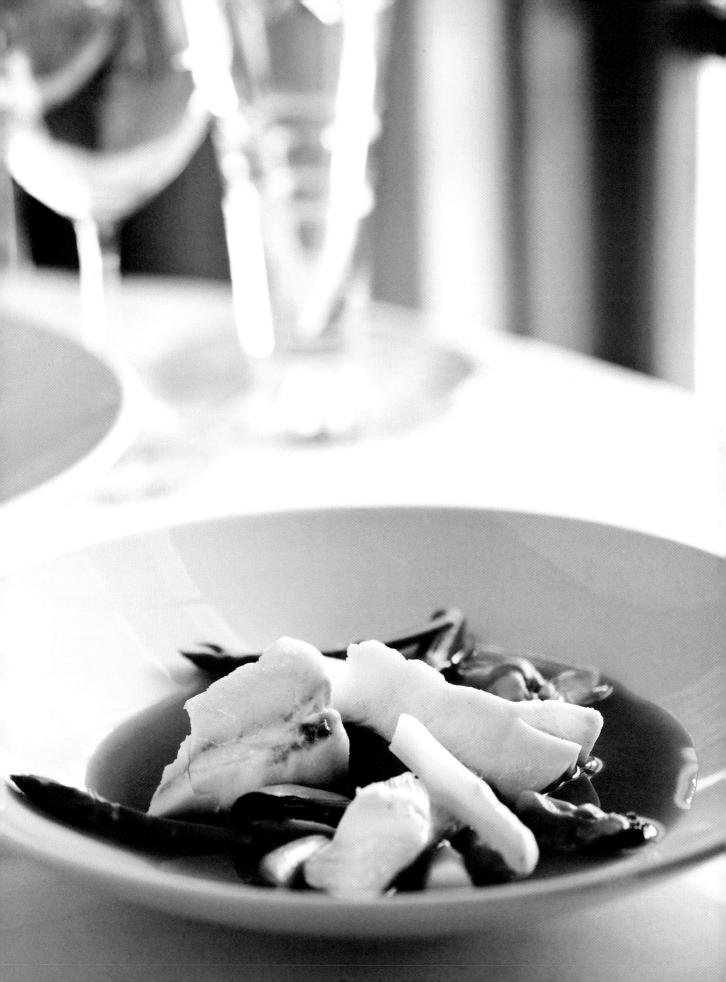

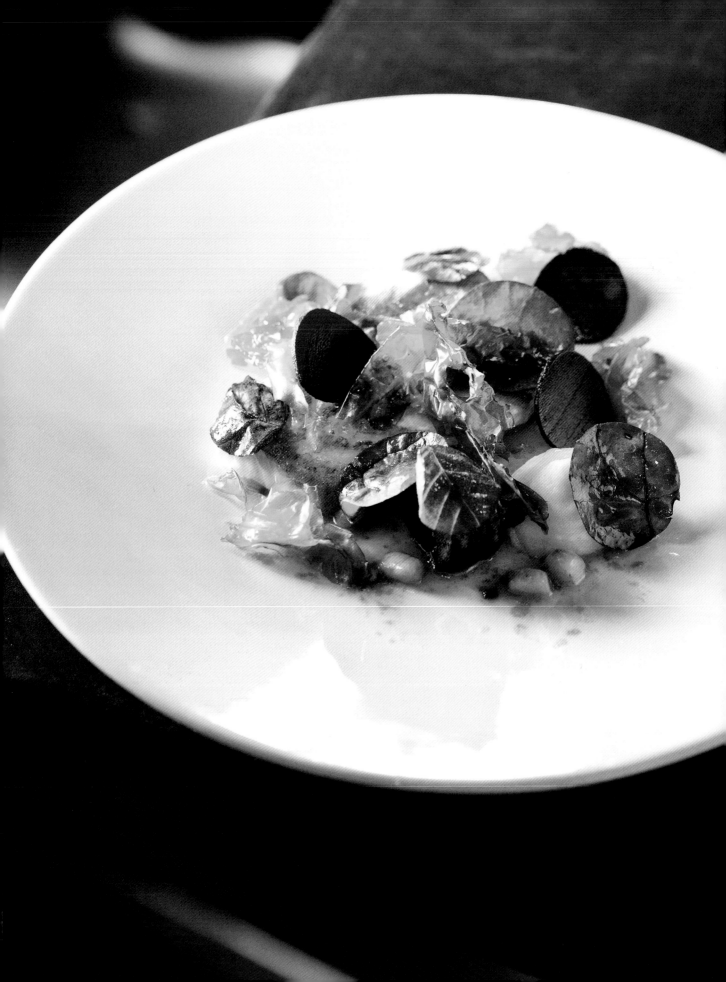

SNAPPER, AMARANTH, SEA LETTUCE, RAINBOW CHARD, SORREL, SQUID

SHANNON BENNETT

COMPONENTS

200 g (7 oz) squid, cleaned

8 cups (2 litres/70 fl oz) chicken stock

lemon zest

sea salt and freshly ground pepper

2 rainbow chard stems, chopped into even lengths

25 ml (1 fl oz) olive oil

handful sea lettuce or baby mache lettuce

4 × 110 g (3¾ oz) snapper fillets, pin-boned

20 g (¾ oz) butter

12 amaranth or baby beetroot (beet) leaves, washed and dried

20 sorrel leaves (see note, page 80)

BEETROOT TERRINE

3 beetroot (beets), peeled

1 tbsp balsamic vinegar

2 thyme sprigs, leaves picked

1 tbsp olive oil

1 tsp salt

POTATO PURÉE

2 large sebago potatoes, peeled

125 g (4½ oz) butter, diced

2½ tbsp milk, warmed

BEETROOT CRUDITÉ

1 large beetroot (beet)

SERVES 4

Preheat oven to 150°C (300°F/Gas 2).

For beetroot terrine, thinly slice beetroot on a mandoline. Whisk balsamic vinegar, thyme, olive oil and salt together in a bowl and add beetroot slices. Layer dressed beetroot slices in a deep baking tin and scatter salt and pepper between each layer. Cover tin with a layer of foil and place a baking tray on top of foil to press. Bake in oven for 35 minutes, or until beetroot is tender. Set aside to cool, then refrigerate until cold.

Combine squid and chicken stock in a large saucepan and braise until tender, about an hour. Strain liquid into a clean saucepan and reduce liquid by half (5–10 minutes) over high heat to desired taste (this is the sauce). Dice braised squid and cook in oil in a frying pan over medium–high heat until crispy. Season with lemon zest and salt and pepper.

For potato purée, cook potatoes in salted boiling water for 25 minutes or until tender. Test potatoes with tip of a knife; if it slides in without resistance, they are cooked. Drain potatoes and allow to steam for a few minutes. Mix potatoes with 50 g (1¾ oz) butter, pass through a food mill, then pass through a fine sieve into a heavy-based saucepan and place over low heat. Using a spatula, beat in rest of butter, one cube at a time. If the mousseline starts to split, add a small amount of warmed milk. Season to taste with salt, place in a piping bag and keep warm until needed.

For beetroot crudité, cut beetroot into 3-cm (1¼-in) circles, then thinly slice on a mandoline. Place in iced water for 5 minutes.

Cook chard in boiling water until tender. Drain well. Heat olive oil in a frying pan, add chard and warm over low heat.

Wash sea lettuce, clean in salted water and dry with paper towel.

Preheat oven to 160°C (315°F/Gas 2–3).

Pan-fry fish in oil for 2 minutes on each side in an ovenproof frying pan, then add 20 g (¾ oz) butter and roast in oven till it is 52°C (125°F) in centre, about 5 minutes. Cut beetroot terrine into 4 portions and reheat in oven while the fish is roasting.

Place a fish fillet on edge of each serving plate and arrange chard over fish. Pipe the potato purée next to fish, place beetroot terrine next to potato, dress with sea lettuce and beetroot crudité, drizzle squid braising liquid around and over fish, sprinkle with squid crisps, amaranth and sorrel leaves.

NOTE: If you can't find sorrel, use frisèe (curly endive) dressed with lemon juice.

DIETITIAN TIP

It's not the potato that's the issue; it is the amount of butter that bumps up the fat and kilojoules.

NIP	WITHOUT POTATO	WITH POTATO
Energy	1301 kJ (311 Cal)	2522 kJ (603 Cal)
Total fat	14 g	40 g
Saturated fat	5 g	22 g
Carbohydrate	10 g	22 g

TASMANIAN SALMON WITH BLACK OLIVE PURÉE ON A BED OF SPRING ONIONS

DANY CHOUET

Simple and delicious, this makes a good main course for summer, served with a green salad and crusty bread.

1 bunch large spring onions (scallions) or 4 white onions, very thinly sliced

2 tbsp extra virgin olive oil, plus 2 tsp for sauce

350 g (12 oz) kalamata olives, pitted

freshly ground pepper

4 Tasmanian salmon fillets, about 200 g (7 oz) each, skin on, pin-boned

1½ tbsp lemon thyme leaves

juice of 1 lemon

SERVES 4

Very gently half cook spring onion or onion in 1 tablespoon extra virgin olive oil in a frying pan over low–medium heat for 5 minutes, without colouring. Purée olives very finely in a food processor with the remaining tablespoon of extra virgin olive oil and a little pepper.

Preheat oven to 210°C (415°F/Gas 6–7).

Season salmon with pepper and sprinkle with thyme, then spread 1½ tablespoons olive purée very carefully onto flesh side of each fillet. Place in a roasting tin, skin side down, surround with spring onion or onion, cover with foil and cook in oven for 8–10 minutes.

When cooked, divide spring onion or onion equally between some warmed serving plates and sit salmon on top.

Deglaze roasting tin with lemon juice, whisk in about 2 teaspoons olive oil, check seasoning, then drizzle over and around salmon.

This recipe is from *So French* by Dany Chouet with Trish Hobbs (Murdoch Books, 2011).

DIETITIAN TIP

As you can see the saturated fat is low, making this dish a good source of polyunsaturated fats. The National Heart Foundation recommends 2–3 serves of oily fish or seafood a week – here is a great way to get a tasty and healthy serve of fish.

NIP

Energy	2367 kJ (566 Cal)
Total fat	32 g
Saturated fat	9 g
Carbohydrate	4 g

LUCA BRASI SLEEPS WITH THE FISHES

AARON HARVIE

I was asked to develop a menu for an Italian–American themed night. There's a famous line from Francis Ford Coppola's 1972 masterpiece The Godfather ... 'Luca Brasi sleeps with the fishes'. This is my take on a classic Italian–American cioppino; it has a little spice and lots of vegetables and seafood.

4 cups (1 litre/35 fl oz) fish stock (homemade or salt-reduced store-bought stock)

12 raw prawns (shrimp), peeled and deveined, heads and shells cleaned and reserved

12 mussels, scrubbed and debearded

12 clams (vongole), scrubbed

12 × 20 g (¾ oz) pieces snapper fillet

TOMATO BASE

1 tbsp olive oil, plus extra for drizzling

2 garlic cloves, roughly chopped

½ onion, roughly chopped

2 carrots, roughly chopped

½ green capsicum (pepper), roughly chopped

1 celery stalk and some leaves, roughly chopped

1 tbsp chopped basil

1 tsp chopped oregano

2 tbsp chopped flat-leaf (Italian) parsley, reserve some to garnish

freshly ground pepper

1 tsp chipotle chilli powder (or normal chilli powder)

2 tbsp white wine

1 tsp Tabasco sauce

1 tbsp red wine vinegar

1 tbsp worcestershire sauce

3 × 400 g (14 oz) tins chopped tomatoes

SERVES 6 WISEGUYS

For tomato base, heat a heavy-based saucepan over medium heat, add olive oil and vegetables and sauté till soft. Add basil, oregano, parsley, pepper, chilli powder, white wine, Tabasco, vinegar and worcestershire sauce and cook until liquid has reduced by half. Finally add tomatoes. Cover, and simmer over low heat for 45 minutes, stirring every 10 minutes, until reduced and thick. Cool in fridge, then blend until puréed. Strain, pressing pulp through sieve, and reserve.

For homemade or store-bought fish stock, heat till almost boiling, reduce to a simmer, add prawn heads and shells. Infuse for 20 minutes. Strain into large saucepan and mix in tomato base.

Bring soup to the boil, reduce heat a little and add mussels, clams and fish. After 4 minutes add prawns, cooking until mussels and clams open. Discard any that do not. Season to taste.

Divide seafood between serving bowls so everyone gets two pieces of everything and ladle soup over. Garnish with some parsley and a drizzle of olive oil.

DIETITIAN TIP
A spicy low-fat recipe from Aaron.

NIP Includes drizzled olive oil when served

Energy	1036 kJ (248 Cal)
Total fat	10 g
Saturated fat	2 g
Carbohydrate	13 g

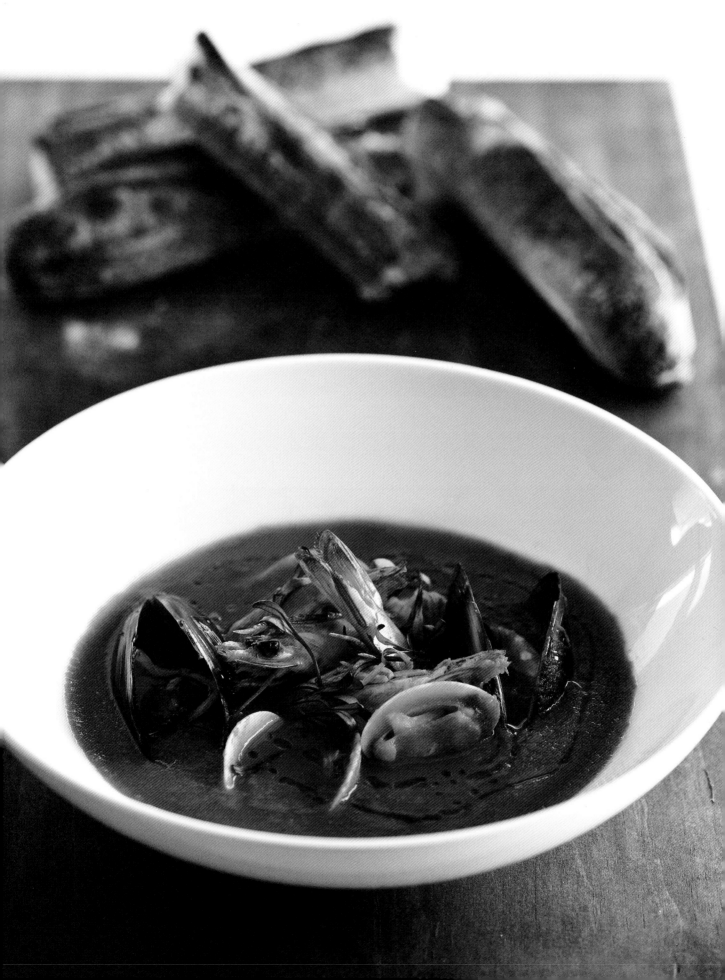

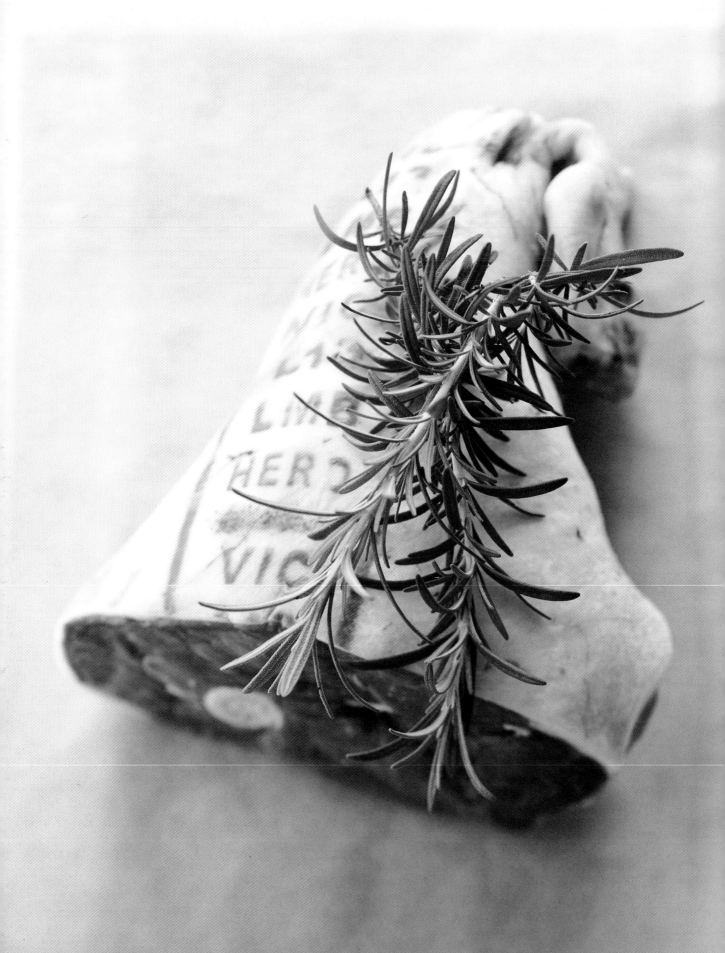

MEAT

LAMB RUMP WITH HUMMUS AND ROASTED CAPSICUM

MATT MORAN

800 g (1 lb 12 oz) lamb rump (2 × 400 g/ 14 oz rumps)

1 knob butter

SPICE RUB

1 tsp coriander (cilantro) seeds

1 tsp cumin seeds

½ tsp smoked paprika

pinch of sea salt

juice of ½ lemon

2½ tbsp olive oil

HUMMUS

200 g (7 oz) dried chickpeas

2 tbsp tahini

juice of ½ lemon

sea salt and freshly ground pepper

100 ml (3½ fl oz) olive oil

ROASTED CAPSICUM

2 red capsicums (peppers)

2½ tbsp olive oil

½ red (Spanish) onion, thinly sliced

2 tsp red wine vinegar

2 tsp chopped flat-leaf (Italian) parsley

SERVES 4

To prepare spice rub, place coriander and cumin seeds in a frying pan over medium heat. Dry-roast spices for 2 minutes until they begin to 'pop'. Transfer seeds to a mortar with smoked paprika, salt, lemon juice and olive oil, then using a pestle grind together to form a paste. Set aside until required.

Trim some fat from lamb rump, then score remaining fat (this will help to render fat while meat is cooking). Rub lamb with prepared spice rub, then leave to marinate in the fridge overnight or for at least 2–3 hours.

To prepare hummus, soak chickpeas in a bowl of water for 12 hours, then drain. Place chickpeas in a large saucepan and cover with cold water. Bring to the boil, then reduce heat to a simmer. Cook chickpeas for 30–40 minutes, or until tender (they should squash easily when pressed). Drain, reserving some cooking liquid. Place chickpeas in a blender with tahini, a squeeze of lemon juice and some salt and pepper. Add a little saved cooking water to assist with consistency, then blend until a smooth paste forms. Continue to blend while you trickle in olive oil in an even stream. Adjust seasoning and lemon juice if desired, then place in fridge until required.

To prepare roasted capsicum, place whole capsicums over a gas flame, turning when required, until skin is charred black. Remove from heat and leave to cool. Scrape away charred skin and remove core and seeds. Cut flesh into 1-cm (½-in) strips, then set aside. Heat olive oil in a frying pan over medium heat and when hot, add onion, season with salt and pepper and cook for

1 minute before adding capsicum strips. Cook for a further 2 minutes before adding vinegar. Cook until vinegar has completely reduced, add parsley, then remove from heat and leave to cool.

Preheat oven to 180°C (350°F/Gas 4).

Heat a frying pan over medium heat and when hot, add butter. Once butter is foaming, add marinated lamb rumps to pan. Cook lamb rumps until brown all over and then place them onto a baking tray. Place tray in oven and roast for 15 minutes. Remove from oven and rest for 10 minutes before serving.

Slice lamb rumps thinly, then serve with hummus and roasted capsicum.

DIETITIAN TIP
Hummus adds fibre and the carbohydrate in this recipe.

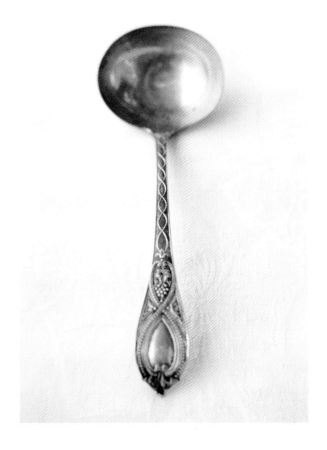

NIP
Energy	3640 kJ (870 Cal)
Total fat	58 g
Saturated fat	13 g
Carbohydrate	24 g

TENDERLOIN STEAK WITH CORIANDER, CUMIN AND LIME

CAROL SELVA RAJAH

This maximum flavour, minimum fuss recipe is guaranteed for success as long as good tenderloin is marinated, grilled, then sliced across the grain quickly. Done this way, beef is the consummate meal that satisfies.

1 cup (200 g/7 oz) basmati rice

2½ cups (625 ml/21½ fl oz) water

pinch of sea salt

500 g (1 lb 2 oz) or 2 pieces beef tenderloin steak

1 tsp cumin seeds, dry roasted and roughly pounded

1 tsp coriander (cilantro) seeds, dry roasted and ground

½ tsp dried chilli flakes

2 tsp good olive oil

2 large handfuls mint leaves

2 tbsp pine nuts

juice of 1 lime

MARINADE

½ tsp lemon zest

2 tbsp lime juice

2 tbsp light soy sauce

DRESSING

1 tbsp balsamic vinegar

2 tbsp lime juice

2 tsp icing (confectioners') sugar

1 kaffir lime leaf, torn

1 tbsp mild chilli sauce

SERVES 4

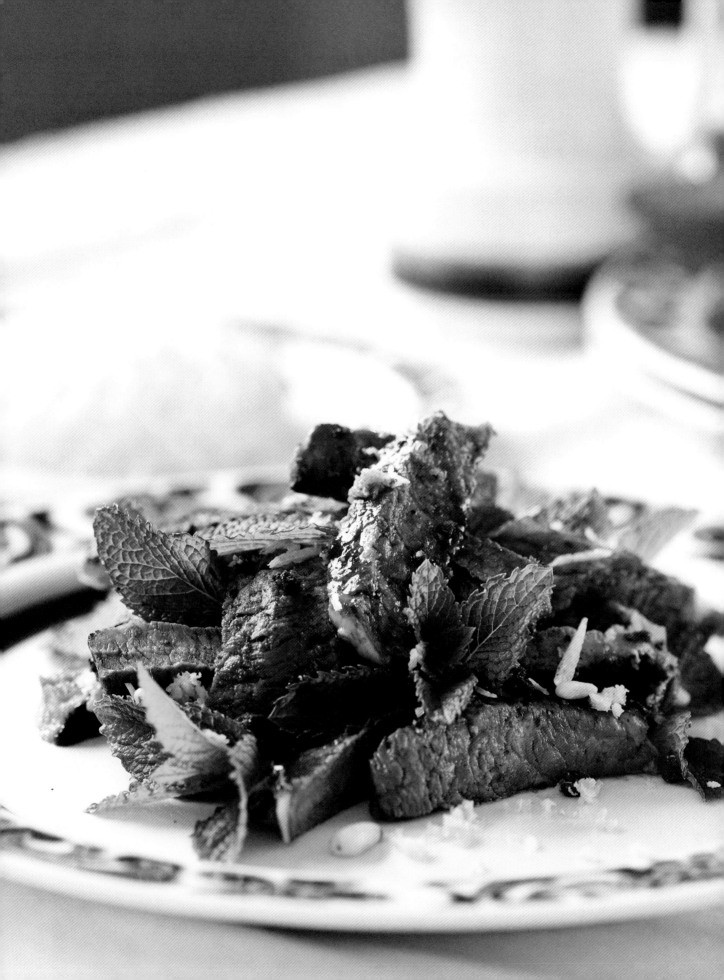

Wash rice in a bowl of water until water is clear. Leave last rinse in the bowl, allowing rice to soak for half an hour. Pour drained rice into a saucepan, add water and salt and bring to the boil. When rice starts to make plopping sounds, after about 10 minutes, turn off heat. Cover pan tightly with a lid, allow rice to cook in its own heat for about 20 minutes. Remove lid, then use chopsticks or a large fork to gently fluff up rice.

Meanwhile, combine all the marinade ingredients, add beef and marinate for about 20 minutes. Remove beef from marinade, then pat dry with paper towel.

Mix cumin, coriander and chilli flakes with olive oil. Rub beef on both sides with spice and oil mixture.

For dressing, combine balsamic vinegar, lime juice, sugar, kaffir lime leaf and chilli sauce and whisk well.

Pour dressing over mint and pine nuts, and toss well.

Preheat grill (broiler) to high. Cook beef on grill, turn over after 2 minutes, then cook for about 2 minutes until medium or well done. Allow beef to rest a minute, then slice it into 2-cm (¾-in) pieces across the grain. Squeeze on a dash of lime.

Scatter mint and pine-nut dressing over beef and serve hot with rice in small portions (or press rice into a small soup bowl and turn out onto serving plates).

DIETITIAN TIP
With the carbohydrate provided by the rice, you need only add a salad to make this low-fat meal complete.

NIP

Energy	1877 kJ (448 Cal)
Total fat	12 g
Saturated fat	3 g
Carbohydrate	40 g

BRAISED ROLLED LAMB LOIN WITH ALMOND STUFFING

RODNEY DUNN

50 g (1¾ oz) butter

1 large onion, finely chopped

½ cup (30 g/1 oz) fresh breadcrumbs

100 g (3½ oz) whole almonds, toasted and coarsely crushed

1 tbsp finely chopped oregano

1 tbsp finely chopped thyme

½ tsp ground cinnamon

sea salt and freshly ground pepper

1.2 kg (2 lb 10 oz) lamb mid-loin, bones and excess fat removed

1 tbsp olive oil

2 cups (500 ml/17 fl oz) chicken stock

1 cinnamon stick

4 allspice berries

SERVES 8

Melt butter in a large frying pan, add onion and sauté over medium heat until softened, 5–6 minutes. Add breadcrumbs, almonds, herbs and ground cinnamon, mix to combine and season to taste with salt and pepper. Remove from heat and set aside to cool.

Preheat oven to 150°C (300°F/Gas 2).

Place lamb, skin side down, on a clean work surface and evenly spread stuffing over loin. Starting at longest side, roll up and secure at 5-cm (2-in) intervals with kitchen twine.

Heat olive oil in a large flameproof casserole dish, add lamb loin and cook over high heat, turning frequently until golden brown, about 5–6 minutes. Add chicken stock and remaining spices and bring to a simmer. Cover, place in oven and cook until meat is tender, 2½–3 hours.

To serve, remove twine, cut lamb into 3-cm (1¼-in) thick slices and serve with a little braising broth.

DIETITIAN TIP
This dish just needs some carbs and vegies to make it a perfect meal.

NIP
Energy   1682 kJ (402 Cal)
Total fat   29 g
Saturated fat   9 g
Carbohydrate   3 g

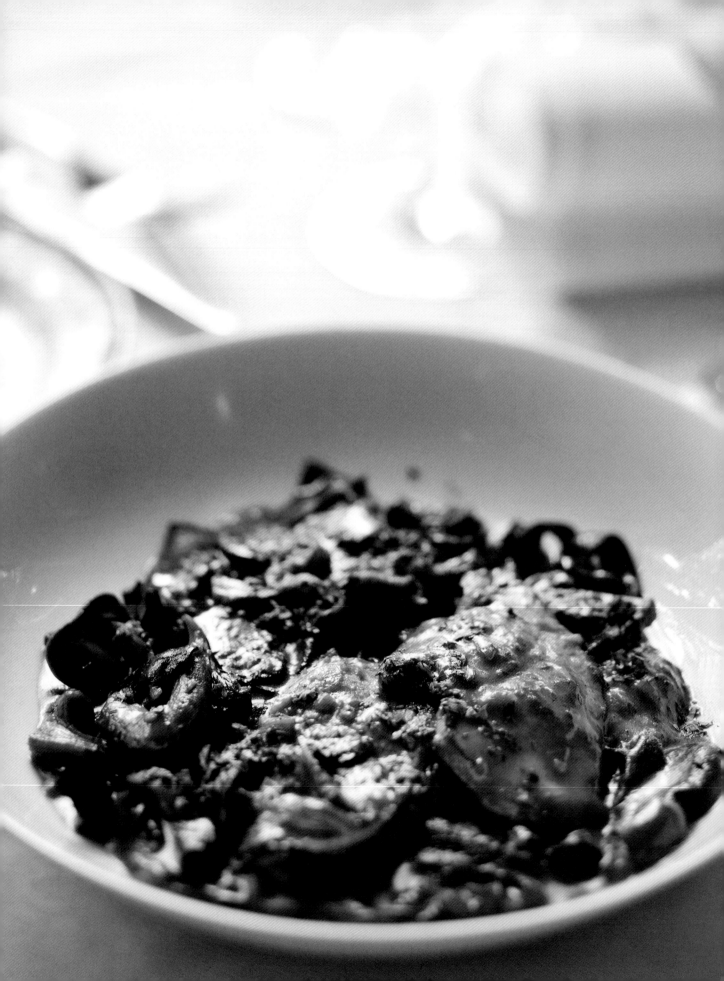

VEAL SCALOPPINE WITH MUSHROOMS

GUY GROSSI

100 g (3½ oz) dried wild mushrooms

200 ml (7 fl oz) olive oil

1 onion, finely chopped

2 garlic cloves, finely chopped

2 bay leaves

45 g (1½ oz) tomato paste (concentrated purée)

100 ml (3½ fl oz) red wine

4 cups (1 litre/35 fl oz) chicken stock

200 g (7 oz) button mushrooms

12 × 50 g (1¾ oz) veal medallions

⅔ cup (100 g/3½ oz) plain (all-purpose) flour

100 ml (3½ fl oz) white wine

100 ml (3½ fl oz) thin (pouring) cream

pinch of sea salt and freshly ground pepper

SERVES 4

Soak dried mushrooms in cold water for 2 hours.

Heat 100 ml (3½ fl oz) olive oil in a saucepan over medium heat. Add onion, garlic and bay leaves and sauté, without colouring, until onion is translucent.

Scoop soaked mushrooms out of water and roughly chop them. Add to onion mixture and sauté for 2 minutes, then add tomato paste and sauté for a further 2 minutes. Deglaze with red wine and simmer for a few minutes before adding stock and button mushrooms. Simmer for 45 minutes while veal is prepared.

Place veal slices between plastic wrap and gently thin out veal with a meat mallet.

In a deep frying pan, heat remaining oil over medium heat. Dust veal in flour and sauté on both sides until golden brown. Deglaze pan with white wine. Ladle in reduced mushroom sauce and add cream. Simmer until well combined and a rich consistency is achieved. Season to taste.

DIETITIAN TIP
Veal is a very lean meat. The high fat content comes from the oil used to sauté the onions and the cream.

NIP
Energy   3402 kJ (813 Cal)
Total fat   59 g
Saturated fat   14 g
Carbohydrate   16 g

RARE ROASTED VENISON, SPICED BEETROOT AND COCONUT SAMBAL

CHRISTINE MANFIELD

3 tbsp vegetable oil

1 tsp sea salt

½ tsp freshly ground pepper

½ tsp garam masala

400 g (14 oz) venison strip loin fillet, trimmed and cut into 4 portions

COCONUT SAMBAL

1 cup (65 g/2½ oz) shredded fresh coconut

3 small green chillies, minced

2 garlic cloves, minced

1 tbsp minced ginger

1 tsp ground turmeric

2 tsp sea salt

120 ml (3¾ fl oz) tamarind water

SPICED BEETROOT

2 tbsp coconut oil

1 tsp sesame oil

2 tbsp fresh curry leaves

4 small green chillies, thinly sliced

1 tsp minced ginger

3 red Asian shallots, thinly sliced

1 tsp ground cumin

4 beetroot (beets), peeled and cut into thin slices

2 tbsp rice or coconut vinegar

2 tsp sea salt

2 tsp caster (superfine) sugar

200 ml (7 fl oz) coconut milk

2 tbsp fresh curry leaves, fried

SERVES 4

To prepare coconut sambal, briefly blend coconut, chilli, garlic, ginger, turmeric and salt in a food processor, just to combine. Add tamarind water and pulse until blended. Set aside at room temperature until ready to serve.

To prepare spiced beetroot, heat both oils in a large saucepan and temper/sauté curry leaves, chilli, ginger and shallot until softened. Stir in cumin and after 20 seconds add beetroot slices. Mix to coat, then add vinegar, salt and sugar, stirring to combine. Fry over high heat, stirring, until beetroot has softened, about 2 minutes. Add coconut milk and cover with lid, reduce heat to low and cook for 15 minutes until beetroot is tender and most juices have been absorbed. Remove from heat, taste and adjust seasoning – it may need a little extra salt. Stir through fried curry leaves.

Mix vegetable oil with salt, pepper and garam masala. Rub spiced oil liberally onto venison portions. Heat a frying pan over high heat and sear venison for 3 minutes, then turn over and cook for a further 2 minutes. Remove from heat and rest meat in pan in a warm place for 5 minutes.

To serve, spoon spiced beetroot onto plates, cut each venison portion into four slices and arrange on top. Garnish with a spoonful of coconut sambal.

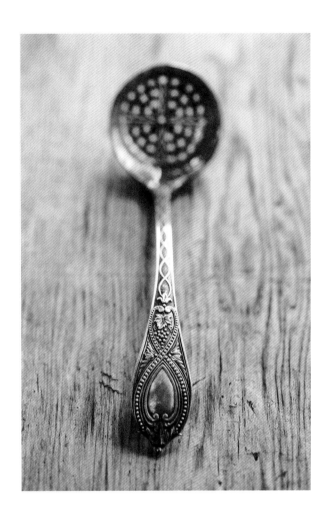

DIETITIAN TIP
The coconut in this recipe is the source of saturated fat. Beware if your cholesterol is high – have this one as a special occasion meal.

NIP
Energy	1783 kJ (426 Cal)
Total fat	28 g
Saturated fat	21 g
Carbohydrate	12 g

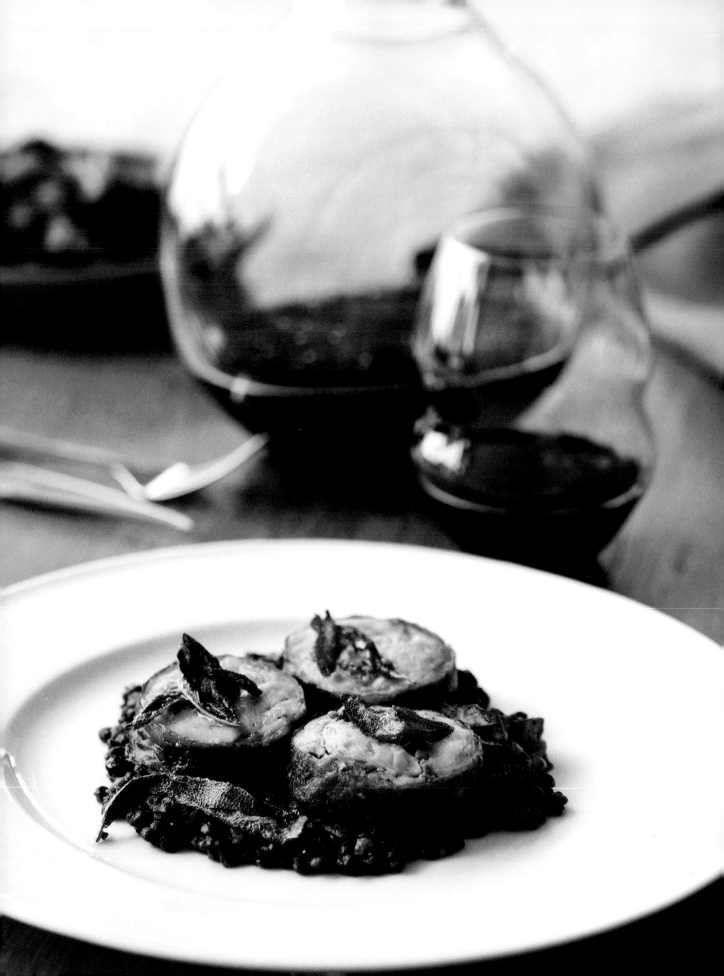

ROAST RABBIT SADDLE
WITH BREAD AND SAGE STUFFING
AND BRAISED LENTILS

STEFANO MANFREDI

1 onion, diced

4 garlic cloves, crushed

100 g (3½ oz) butter

2½ cups (150 g/5½ oz) fresh breadcrumbs

50 g (1¾ oz) Italian mustard fruit, thinly sliced

¾ cup (100 g/3½ oz) parmesan cheese, grated

4 tbsp chopped flat-leaf (Italian) parsley

4 tbsp chopped sage leaves

sea salt and freshly ground pepper

8 slices prosciutto

2 farmed rabbit saddles (approx. 1.5 kg/ 3 lb 5 oz in total), each carefully boned as one whole piece

2 tbsp extra virgin olive oil

BRAISED LENTILS

½ celery heart, finely chopped

1 carrot, finely chopped

1 onion, finely chopped

1 leek, sliced into half rounds about 5-mm (¼ -in) thick

2 garlic cloves, minced

⅓ cup (80 ml/2½ fl oz) extra virgin olive oil

4 tbsp roughly chopped flat-leaf (Italian) parsley

1 rosemary sprig, chopped

1 thyme sprig, chopped

500 g (1 lb 2 oz) Puy or tiny blue-green lentils, washed well

4 cups (1 litre/35 fl oz) vegetable or chicken stock

200 g (7 oz) tomato passata (puréed tomatoes)

SERVES 6

To make stuffing, lightly fry onion and garlic in butter until soft but not coloured. Take from heat and add to breadcrumbs, mustard fruit, parmesan, parsley, half the sage, salt and pepper. Mix well and let it cool down.

Lay prosciutto slices flat on a clean board or kitchen bench in two sets of four so each slice is slightly overlapping previous one. Put one rabbit saddle on first set of four prosciutto slices and other saddle on next set. Distribute stuffing evenly in middle of each saddle, making sure stuffing is just enough to roll (too much will be difficult to hold). Roll up so that prosciutto covers rabbit completely in a tight sausage. Wrap tightly in plastic wrap and set in fridge for 2–3 hours.

An hour before serving, take rolled rabbit out of fridge to reach room temperature.

Preheat oven to 200°C (400°F/Gas 6). Remove plastic wrap and lay rabbit rolls in a roasting tin. Sprinkle olive oil over surface of each roll. Add remaining sage leaves, season with salt and pepper. Roast for 15–20 minutes. Test by inserting a skewer into centre of roll. Rabbit is cooked if juice flows clear without blood. Remove from the oven and rest for 10 minutes before slicing and serving with braised lentils.

For braised lentils, in a large saucepan, lightly fry vegetables and garlic in olive oil for a few minutes without colouring them. Add parsley, rosemary and thyme and continue to cook for another minute or two. Add lentils and stir. Add stock and tomato passata till lentils are covered. Simmer for 30–50 minutes till lentils are tender. Add more liquid if they are too dry as they cook. Season with salt and pepper to taste.

DIETITIAN TIP

Like all game, rabbit is a lean meat. The lentils add lots of fibre.

NIP

Energy	3854 kJ (921 Cal)
Total fat	48 g
Saturated fat	18 g
Carbohydrate	54 g

SOFRITO

JONATHAN BARTHELMESS

Veal in garlic with wine and parsley sauce – a specialty from the Greek
island of Corfu. It is said that a good sofrito is made from very few ingredients but
it is the quality of the ingredients that shines through. This dish varies from
house to house – this is my version based on the recipes I have found.

2 large brown onions, diced

165 ml (5¼ fl oz) extra virgin olive oil

4 × 150 g (5½ oz) pieces veal fillet

plain (all-purpose) flour, for dusting

4 garlic cloves, thinly sliced

½ bunch flat-leaf (Italian) parsley, very
roughly chopped

1 bay leaf

sea salt and freshly ground pepper

1 cup (250 ml/9 fl oz) white wine

½ cup (125 ml/4 fl oz) chicken stock

SERVES 4

Place onion and 2 tablespoons olive oil in a
saucepan over low heat, half cover with lid
and cook for 20 minutes until very soft but not
coloured.

Slice each piece of veal into 4 pieces across
the grain. Bash meat out flat with a meat mallet
and dust with flour.

Heat remaining olive oil in a heavy-based
frying pan until hot enough for veal to sizzle and
shallow-fry veal for a few seconds on each side.
Remove and set aside.

Remove excess oil from pan. Add garlic
and cook over medium heat until just coloured,
then add parsley, bay leaf and cooked onion.
Season with salt and pepper, add white wine and
increase heat to high. Reduce until parsley and
garlic start to fry. Add chicken stock and reduce
to a sauce consistency. Taste and season. Add
cooked veal to sauce and warm through, then
serve on plates.

DIETITIAN TIP
Make sure the oil is very hot before adding the
veal, as this will limit the amount of fat that will
be absorbed into the flour.

NIP
Energy   1920 kJ (459 Cal)
Total fat   30 g
Saturated fat   5 g
Carbohydrate   5 g

LAMB NECK FILLET WITH QUINOA AND HAZELNUTS

DETLEF HAUPT

Lamb neck fillet is very versatile, and it's a cheap but very tasty cut of meat.
I usually use neck fillets in curries and casseroles but this is something different
and slightly posher. This would also work with other cuts of meat.

LAMB NECK FILLET

2 × 150–170 g (5½–6 oz) lamb neck fillets

sea salt and freshly ground pepper

1 garlic clove, crushed

1 tbsp chopped rosemary

1 tbsp mashed anchovy fillets

1⅔ cups (100 g/3½ oz) fresh breadcrumbs

1 egg yolk

2 tbsp olive oil

1 tbsp extra virgin olive oil

sprigs fresh marjoram

TRUSS TOMATOES

8 baby truss tomatoes

2 tbsp olive oil

QUINOA AND HAZELNUTS

210 ml (7½ fl oz) good-quality chicken stock

2 tbsp olive oil

120 g (4¼ oz) quinoa, rinsed and drained

35 g (1¼ oz) unsalted butter

30 g (1 oz) Australian hazelnuts, uniformly crushed

CAPONATA VEGETABLES

30 g (1 oz) diced onion

100 ml (3½ fl oz) olive oil

80 g (2¾ oz) diced eggplant (aubergine)

50 g (1¾ oz) diced red capsicum (pepper)

50 g (1¾ oz) diced yellow capsicum (pepper)

50 g (1¾ oz) diced fleshy tomato skins

1 tbsp baby basil leaves

1 tbsp anchovy essence

CARAMELISED SHALLOTS

15 g (½ oz) unsalted butter

2 French shallots, peeled

1 tbsp brown sugar

1 tbsp balsamic vinegar

SERVES 4

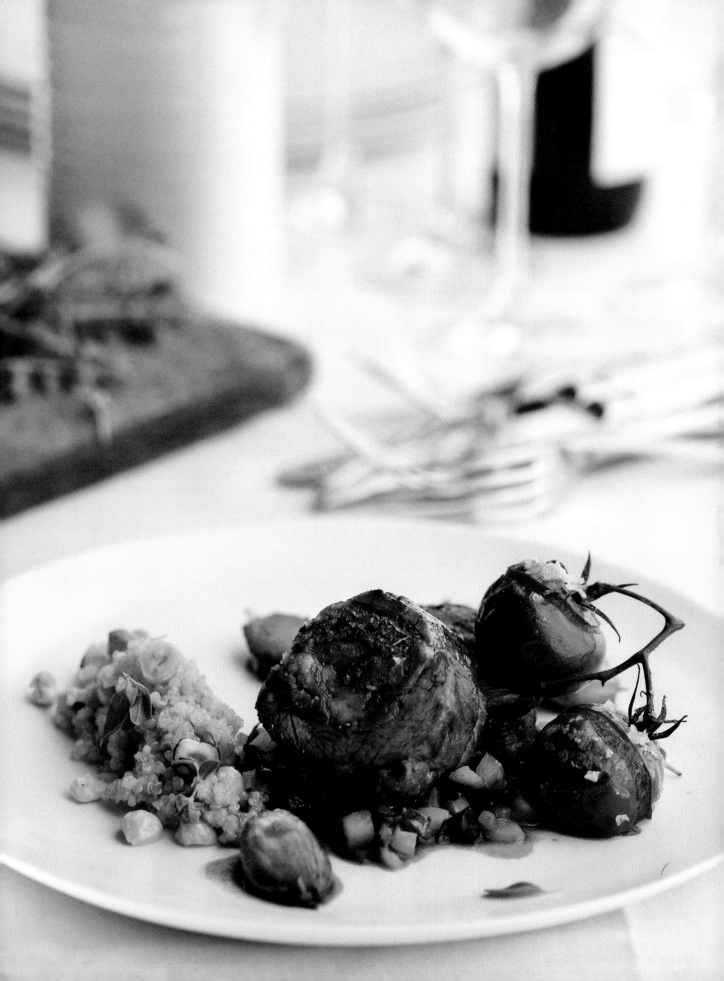

Preheat oven to 180°C (350°F/Gas 4).

For lamb neck fillet, with a sharp knife, slit each fillet open but don't cut all the way through. Season well on both sides, flatten meat slightly if necessary. Mix garlic, rosemary, mashed anchovy and breadcrumbs, add egg yolk to bind and divide the mixture in half, placing a portion in centre of each piece of meat. Roll up meat and secure with kitchen twine (not too tight). Season well on all sides. Heat olive oil in an ovenproof frying pan over low heat and brown meat on all sides. Place in oven, cook to medium, about 8 minutes, and let rest, covered with foil in a warm place.

For truss tomatoes, toss tomatoes in olive oil and sprinkle with salt. Place in oven and roast until skin is blistered, about 3–5 minutes.

For quinoa and hazelnuts, bring chicken stock and olive oil to the boil in a saucepan. Using a fork, sprinkle quinoa into stock, stirring so it will absorb all the liquid. Turn off heat once quinoa has absorbed all the stock, about 3–4 minutes. Cover and let quinoa steam for 5–10 minutes. Before serving, fold in butter and sprinkle with hazelnuts.

For caponata vegetables, sauté onion in a frying pan over low heat with plenty of olive oil until translucent. Add eggplant and sauté for a few minutes, add capsicums and tomato skins, and cook until all combined, approximately 3 minutes. Stir in basil and anchovy essence, season with salt and pepper and set aside. The vegetables should look colourful, appetising and loose, not sticking together.

For caramelised shallots, melt butter in an ovenproof frying pan, add shallots and sprinkle with brown sugar and balsamic vinegar. Ensure shallots are evenly coated. Place pan in oven and let shallots caramelise for 10–20 minutes.

To serve, use a sharp knife to remove twine from lamb neck fillets, and cut lamb into slices. Place a few tablespoonfuls of quinoa and hazelnuts on each plate. Dress a few tablespoonfuls of caponata vegetables around quinoa. Place meat on top of quinoa. Garnish with roasted truss tomatoes, drizzle with lamb jus, place a couple of caramelised shallots on top and finally add a drizzle of extra virgin olive oil and some sprigs of fresh marjoram.

DIETITIAN TIP
Lamb fillet is a lean meat. The fat in this recipe is mostly from the oil and butter added during the cooking. Quinoa is a high-protein grain that is also a good source of carbohydrate.

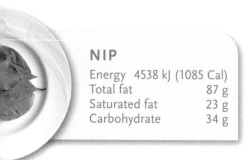

NIP
Energy 4538 kJ (1085 Cal)	
Total fat	87 g
Saturated fat	23 g
Carbohydrate	34 g

VENISON TENDERLOIN WITH RED WINE SAUCE

MICHAEL MANNERS

700–800 g (1 lb 9 oz–1 lb 12 oz) Mandagery Creek venison tenderloin

1 tbsp redcurrant jelly

70 g (2½ oz) prunes, pitted

zest and juice of 1 orange

SPICE RUB

1 tsp crushed black peppercorns

1 tsp allspice berries

1 blade of mace

5-cm (2-in) cinnamon stick

2 tsp coriander (cilantro) seeds

1 tbsp juniper berries

75 ml (2¼ fl oz) olive oil

MARINADE

400 g (14 oz) onion, thinly sliced

1 carrot, diced

½ single celery stalk, cut into small dice

30–40 ml (1–1¼ fl oz) lightly flavoured olive oil

1 bay leaf

230 ml (7¾ fl oz) red wine

450 ml (16 fl oz) good-quality beef stock

TO SERVE

mashed potato

glazed carrot

SERVES 4

For spice rub, grind peppercorns, allspice, mace, cinnamon, coriander seeds and juniper berries and mix well with oil.

Rub half the spice rub onto meat and set aside.

For marinade, sweat onion, carrot and celery in oil in a saucepan over medium heat until cooked and lightly caramelised. Add remaining spice rub and bay leaf, and deglaze with red wine. Reduce by half, add beef stock and cook gently for 15 minutes. Allow to cool. Add venison to marinade and marinate overnight in fridge.

Next day, remove meat from marinade and dry well. Reserve marinade. Preheat oven to 200°C (400°F/Gas 6).

Heat a large ovenproof frying pan over medium–high heat and sear meat on all sides. Transfer to oven and roast for 6–10 minutes until rare but no more than medium-rare. Allow to rest in a warm place.

While the meat is resting, make the red wine sauce. Pour marinade into a saucepan and simmer until reduced by half. Add redcurrant jelly, prunes and orange zest and juice, and reduce to a sauce-like consistency, about 4–5 minutes.

Serve venison with red wine sauce, mashed potato and glazed carrot.

DIETITIAN TIP
Venison is a very lean meat. The carbohydrate in this recipe essentially comes from the prunes and juice.

NIP Excludes mashed potato and glazed carrot

Energy	1754 kJ (419 Cal)
Total fat	18 g
Saturated fat	4 g
Carbohydrate	21 g

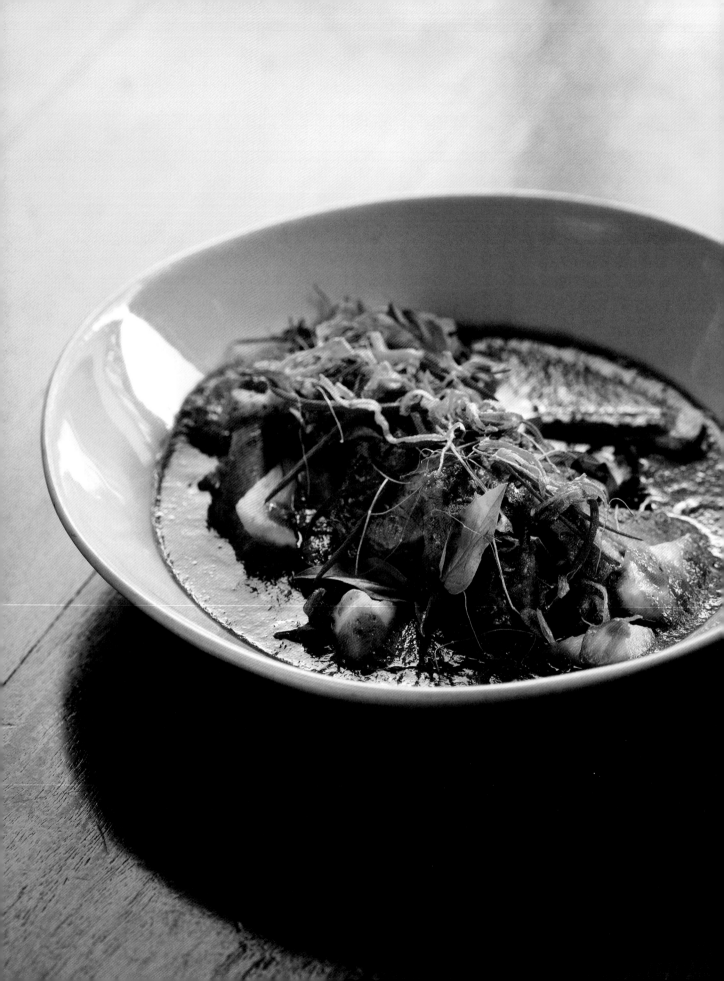

PINEAPPLE CURRY OF GRILLED PORK

MARTIN BOETZ

1 × 400 g (14 oz) piece pork neck, rubbed with fennel seeds and sea salt

1 cup (250 ml/9 fl oz) coconut cream

100 g (3½ oz) palm sugar (jaggery), shaved

100 ml (3½ fl oz) fish sauce

¼ pineapple, peeled and chopped into spoon- and fork-sized pieces

3 long red chillies, halved and seeded

6 kaffir lime leaves

2 cups (500 ml/17 fl oz) coconut milk

20 g (¾ oz) Thai basil leaves

CURRY PASTE

5 large dried red chillies

2 tbsp finely chopped French shallots

3 tbsp finely diced garlic

1 tbsp finely chopped lemongrass, white part only

3 slices galangal

1 tbsp diced coriander (cilantro) root

1 tbsp kaffir lime zest

50 g (1¾ oz) smoked river trout

1 tbsp white peppercorns

1 tsp sea salt

1 tsp fennel seeds

SERVES 4

Grill (broil) pork over medium heat for about 10–12 minutes on each side, then allow to rest for another 10–12 minutes. You can also grill the pork on the barbecue.

Make curry paste by pounding ingredients using a mortar and pestle to a uniform paste. To refine, put in a food processor and process until very fine.

Heat coconut cream in a frying pan over medium heat until it separates, add curry paste and cook until fragrant. Season with palm sugar and fish sauce. Add pineapple, chilli and lime leaves and continue to cook out curry paste on a low–medium heat until it is fragrant and the rawness cannot be detected, about 8–10 minutes. Moisten with coconut milk, check seasoning: it should be sweet, salty and slightly sour.

Slice pork, add it to the cooked curry, then stir in basil. Do not cook pork for any longer. To serve, garnish with chilli julienne, lime leaf julienne and fried eschallots (optional).

DIETITIAN TIP
The carbohydrate in this meal comes from the palm sugar. If you are taking insulin, adjust accordingly – others beware.

NIP
Energy   2466 kJ (589 Cal)
Total fat   37 g
Saturated fat   30 g
Carbohydrate   32 g

YOUNG GOAT, BLOOD ORANGES AND MYRTLE WITH BURGHUL AND POMEGRANATE PILAU

GEORGE BIRON

Young goat is sweet and delicate without any overt 'sheepy' flavours. It is best if hung for about 3 weeks before roasting. Young goat is available from Italian, Vietnamese or halal butchers and they will hang it for you on request. For ease of carving, have the butcher bone it for you. But you can leave it on the bone for a more rustic and flavourful result.

Myrtle is a useful garden plant and very common in Sardinian cooking. It has small purple berries that have a taste similar to juniper berries. They impart a wonderful exotic flavour to meats while roasting. Substitute juniper berries and bay leaves if you have difficulty in finding myrtle. The myrtle is not eaten; it is used to exhale its wonderful aroma to the dish, which can be served covered with the myrtle but removed as it's being carved.

1.5 kg (3 lb 5 oz) well-hung young goat forequarter or long leg

1 tbsp olive oil

3 garlic cloves, crushed

1 bunch myrtle leaves or 10 juniper berries

VEGETABLE BASE

100 g (3½ oz) chopped onion

35 g (1¼ oz) green garlic, sliced (see note)

6 blood oranges, peeled and sliced

50 g (1¾ oz) carrot, chopped

50 g (1¾ oz) celery, chopped

100 ml (3½ fl oz) olive oil

sea salt and freshly ground pepper

PILAU

1 tsp myrtle leaves or juniper berries

1 tsp fennel seeds

1 tsp cardamom seeds

1 tsp ground cinnamon

a little red or green chilli, thinly sliced

2 tsp sea salt

2½ tbsp olive oil

100 g (3½ oz) diced onion

250 g (9 oz) coarse burghul (bulgur)

2 cups (500 ml/17 fl oz) water

seeds of 2 pomegranates

SERVES 6

One day before cooking, rub goat with olive oil and crushed garlic. Place in the fridge overnight.

Preheat oven to 160°C (315°F/Gas 2–3).

For vegetable base, mix onion, garlic, orange, carrot, celery and oil in a roasting tin and season with salt and pepper.

Lay goat on vegetable base and cover with myrtle leaves or juniper berries. Roast slowly for about 2 hours till well coloured and very tender. Rest in a warm place for 15 minutes. Discard myrtle or berries just before serving.

For pilau, combine myrtle or juniper berries, fennel seeds, cardamom, cinnamon, chilli and salt in a saucepan over low heat and fry in olive oil until fragrant. Add onion and 250 g (9 oz) vegetable base from roasted goat. Mix with burghul, add water and cook slowly, covered, for 20 minutes till burghul is soft and fluffy. Sprinkle pomegranate seeds on top – do not mix them in or they will lose their cool refreshing flavour.

Slice the goat and serve the pilau as a side dish.

NOTE: Green garlic is young garlic with the green stem attached.

DIETITIAN TIP

As an accompaniment to this meal, burghul is a high-fibre alternative to rice. It's quite low in fat too.

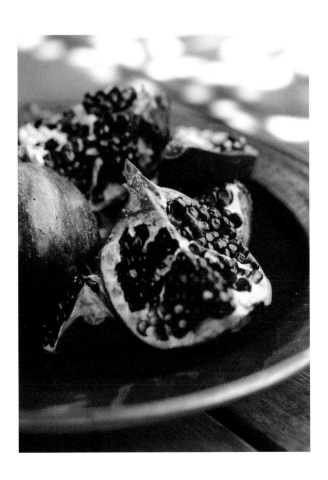

NIP

Energy	2516 kJ (601 Cal)
Total fat	21 g
Saturated fat	4 g
Carbohydrate	40 g

WARM ORIENTAL DUCK
AND MANGO SALAD

LUKE MANGAN

2 duck breasts (120–150 g/4¼–5½ oz each), skin and bones removed

1 tsp Chinese five spice

1 tsp sunflower oil

DRESSING

2 tbsp lime juice

1 tsp fish sauce

1 tbsp soy sauce

2 tsp clear honey

SALAD

120 g (4¼ oz) baby salad leaves (mesclun)

1 small mango, cut into matchsticks

150 g (5½ oz) bean sprouts

1 red (Spanish) onion, thinly sliced

1 handful mint leaves

1 tbsp sesame seeds, toasted

SERVES 2

Slice duck into 1-cm (½-in) wide strips and toss with Chinese five spice.

Heat oil in a wok or frying pan over medium–high heat and stir-fry duck for 2 minutes, or until nicely browned but still pink in the middle. Transfer to a large bowl and stir in combined dressing ingredients. Set aside to cool to room temperature.

To serve, combine salad leaves with mango, bean sprouts and duck mixture. Top with onion, mint and sesame seeds.

DIETITIAN TIP
As duck is a higher fat meat than chicken, removing the skin, as Luke suggests, lowers the fat content significantly.

NIP

Energy	1366 kJ (326 Cal)
Total fat	14 g
Saturated fat	3 g
Carbohydrate	16 g

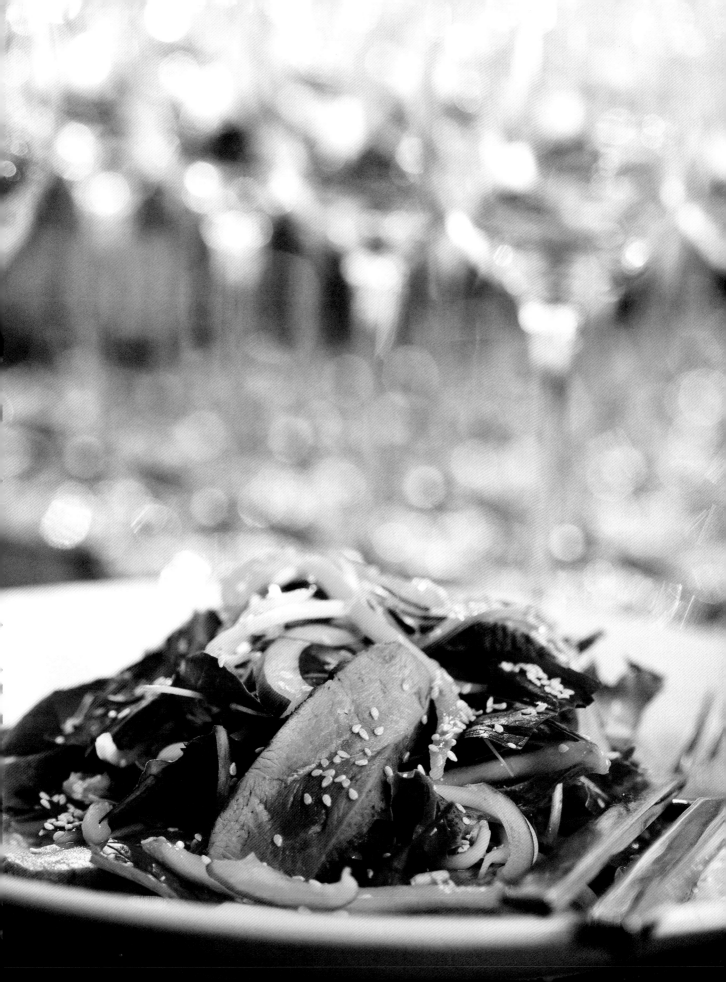

ROASTED CHICKEN AND GREEN AND WHITE ASPARAGUS WITH PARSLEY AND GARLIC EMULSION

GUILLAUME BRAHIMI

1 tbsp olive oil

4 free-range boneless chicken breasts, skin on

8 green asparagus spears, peeled and trimmed

8 white asparagus spears, peeled and trimmed

2½ tbsp water

125 g (4½ oz) butter, cut into 1-cm (½-in) dice

⅓ cup (80 ml/2½ fl oz) chicken jus (see brown chicken stock recipe opposite)

PARSLEY AND GARLIC EMULSION

25 garlic cloves, peeled

200 ml (7 fl oz) brown chicken stock (see recipe following)

120 ml (3¾ fl oz) thin (pouring) cream

1 bunch flat-leaf (Italian) parsley, leaves only

SERVES 4

For parsley and garlic emulsion, place garlic and chicken stock in a small saucepan over medium heat, cover and cook for 30 minutes, or until garlic is soft. Pour in 100 ml (3½ fl oz) cream, bring back to the boil, then remove pan from heat. Bring a saucepan of water to the boil, add parsley and cook for 1 minute. Remove parsley leaves with a slotted spoon and transfer to a bowl of iced water. Remove parsley and squeeze out all excess water. Place garlic and stock in a blender with parsley and blend until smooth. Pass mixture through a fine sieve and set aside in fridge to chill as quickly as possible.

Preheat oven to 180°C (350°F/Gas 4).

Place a large frying pan over medium heat, add oil and when hot, add chicken breasts, skin side down. Reduce heat to low–medium, then cook for 4 minutes, or until golden brown. Turn chicken over and seal other side for 1 minute. Transfer chicken breasts, skin side up, to a baking tray and roast in oven for 13 minutes, or until cooked. Remove from oven and set aside to rest in a warm place for 10 minutes before serving.

Bring a saucepan of salted water to the boil. Cook green asparagus for 2 minutes, remove with a slotted spoon and place in a bowl of iced water. Cook white asparagus in same boiling water for 2½ minutes and place in iced water with green asparagus. Drain well.

Heat water in a large saucepan over low heat. Add diced butter, one piece at a time, whisking until combined. Once all butter is incorporated, add asparagus and toss to coat and heat through.

Bring chicken jus to the boil in a small saucepan. Gently reheat parsley and garlic emulsion in another saucepan. Lightly whip remaining 20 ml (½ fl oz) cream and fold into emulsion.

To serve, slice each chicken breast into three pieces and place on a serving plate. Arrange asparagus on top. Pour boiling chicken jus over asparagus, and spoon on parsley and garlic emulsion. Serve immediately.

BROWN CHICKEN STOCK

2 tbsp olive oil

2 kg (4 lb 8 oz) chicken wings, roughly chopped into 2-cm (¾-in) pieces

1 onion, roughly cut into 2-cm (¾-in) dice

1 celery stalk, roughly cut into 2-cm (¾-in) dice

1 carrot, roughly cut into 2-cm (¾-in) dice

½ garlic head, or 1 garlic head cut in half across the middle

¼ bunch thyme

1 bay leaf

4 litres (140 fl oz) water

MAKES 8 CUPS (2 LITRES/70 FL OZ)

For brown chicken stock, heat 1 tablespoon olive oil in a large saucepan over high heat. Add half the chicken and cook, without stirring, for 3–4 minutes. Continue to cook, stirring constantly, for about 5 minutes or until chicken is very brown all over, then remove from pan. Add remaining oil to pan and repeat process with remaining chicken. Place onion, celery, carrot and garlic in the same pan and cook, stirring occasionally,

for 6–8 minutes, or until soft and coloured. Return chicken to pan, add herbs and stir to combine. Pour in water and bring to the boil, skimming off top layer of fat. Reduce heat and simmer, occasionally skimming the top, for 4 hours to release all the flavour from the meat and vegetables. Strain stock through a fine sieve and chill immediately. Store in fridge for up to 3 days or freeze for up to 1 month.

For chicken jus, pour all brown chicken stock into a saucepan and place over medium heat. Cook for about 1 hour, regularly skimming the top, until reduced to 650 ml (22½ fl oz). Strain through a fine sieve before using.

DIETITIAN TIP
This recipe is calculated as each chicken breast weighing 150 g (5 ½ oz) (skin on). The fat content is higher when you leave the skin on the chicken. For the lowest fat version of this dish, remove the skin before cooking, but be aware that the chicken may dry out more during cooking.

NIP
Energy   2526 kJ (604 Cal)
Total fat   53 g
Saturated fat   28 g
Carbohydrate   5 g

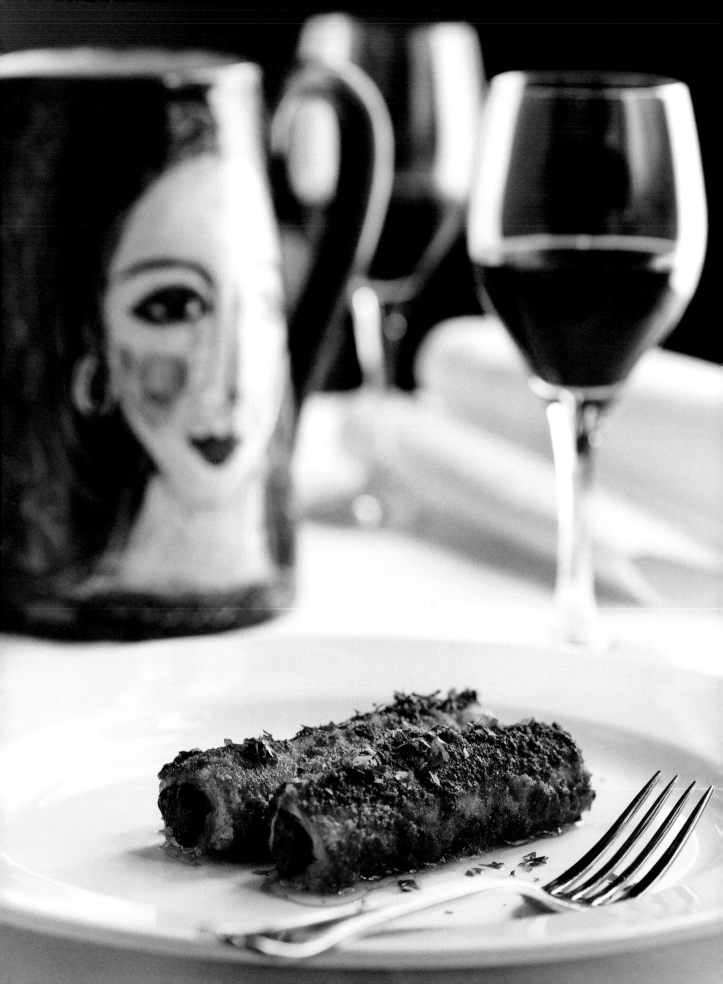

BRACIOLETTE REGINALDO

CRUMBED VEAL ROLL WITH SPINACH, NUTMEG AND PARMESAN

ARMANDO PERCUOCO

1 kg (2 lb 4 oz) baby English spinach leaves

220 g (7¾ oz) unsalted butter

1 whole nutmeg, freshly grated, or
5 tsp freshly grated nutmeg

salt, to taste

180 g (6½ oz) parmesan cheese, finely grated

8 thin slices veal scaloppine

1⅔ cups (300 g/10½ oz) dry breadcrumbs

100 ml (3½ fl oz) vegetable oil

3 tbsp lemon juice

2½ tbsp extra virgin olive oil

1 tbsp finely chopped flat-leaf (Italian) parsley

SERVES 4

Add water to a saucepan large enough to hold spinach and bring to the boil. Add spinach, push down with a spoon, and blanch for 40 seconds, stirring to cook evenly. Strain and refresh under cold running water. Turn to refresh evenly.

Squeeze spinach to remove water (or spinach farce or stuffing won't set).

Place a saucepan over low–medium heat, add butter, nutmeg and salt, and melt to thoroughly combine. Add spinach and mix together for 2 minutes over medium heat. Add 100 g (3½ oz) parmesan and mix. Remove to a tray and cool in the fridge to set and harden.

Once spinach farce is hardened and cool, form logs about 2 cm (¾ in) wide, the same length as the veal slices. Lay out veal slices and sprinkle each with remaining parmesan. Place a spinach log at one end of each veal slice and roll up to form a tight, firm roll. This step can be done beforehand. Cover veal rolls in plastic wrap and leave in fridge until needed.

Preheat cooktop or barbecue hotplate to medium–hot.

Set breadcrumbs and 50 ml (1¾ fl oz) vegetable oil in two separate trays. Push each veal roll into breadcrumbs. Transfer to vegetable oil to lightly coat, then return to breadcrumbs to coat evenly.

Drizzle a little vegetable oil on hotplate, lay down all veal rolls, then drizzle more oil between each roll and cook until you see breadcrumbs starting to go golden brown. Turn. Keep cooking and turning, removing any loose burnt breadcrumbs, until all sides are golden brown, about 6–7 minutes.

Place cooked braciolette on a board and cut off rough ends. Plate two per person.

In a small bowl, combine lemon juice, extra virgin olive oil and a pinch of salt and mix together with a fork. Drizzle over braciolette and sprinkle with parsley.

DIETITIAN TIP
The high saturated fat content comes from the butter and parmesan cheese, so go easy if you have high cholesterol.

NIP

Energy	5734 kJ (1370 Cal)
Total fat	90 g
Saturated fat	44 g
Carbohydrate	53 g

GRILLED LAMB RUMP, SAUTÉED POTATOES, CHERRY TOMATOES, BEANS AND SALTED RICOTTA

PHILIP JOHNSON

6 × 180–200 g (6½–7 oz) lamb rumps, trimmed, leaving a little fat

1 tbsp olive oil

sea salt and freshly ground pepper

6 large southern gold potatoes (or similar), steamed in their skins, cut into thick slices

40 g (1½ oz) unsalted butter

100 g (3½ oz) green beans, trimmed

100 g (3½ oz) yellow beans, trimmed

3–4 tbsp herb mayonnaise (see following recipe)

200 g (7 oz) semi-dried (sun-blushed) cherry tomatoes

250 g (9 oz) salted ricotta cheese

beef or veal jus, demi-glace or veal glaze, warmed, to serve (available from good delicatessens)

SERVES 6

Preheat oven to 180°C (350°F/Gas 4).

Brush lamb rumps with olive oil and season with salt and pepper. Heat a large heavy-based frying pan over high heat. Seal lamb on both sides until well coloured, then transfer to a baking tray and roast in oven for 10–12 minutes. Alternatively, seal and cook lamb on a barbecue. Rest in a warm place for 5 minutes.

Heat a heavy-based frying pan over medium heat. Sauté potato slices in butter until golden, turning to colour both sides.

Steam or boil beans in salted boiling water until tender, drain. Toss with herb mayonnaise and season lightly with salt and pepper.

To serve, put potato slices in the centre of serving plates. Arrange beans over potatoes, then place 3–4 cherry tomatoes around plate. Grate salted ricotta over beans. Slice lamb rumps into 4–5 slices, then arrange over top. Drizzle warm jus around plate.

HERB MAYONNAISE

2 egg yolks

1 tbsp dijon mustard

1 small handful basil leaves

1 small handful flat-leaf (Italian) parsley leaves

3 tbsp snipped chives

juice of ½ lemon

1 cup (250 ml/9 fl oz) vegetable oil

3 tbsp extra virgin olive oil

sea salt and freshly ground pepper

MAKES ABOUT 1½ CUPS (375 ML/13 FL OZ)

Put egg yolks, mustard, herbs and lemon juice in a food processor and blend until smooth. With machine running, slowly drizzle in combined oils until mayonnaise is well blended and thick. You may need to thin mayonnaise with a little hot water. Season with salt and pepper. If you need to adjust acidity, add extra lemon juice. Herb mayonnaise will keep for 1–2 weeks when stored, refrigerated, in an airtight container, and can be used as a salad dressing or spread.

DIETITIAN TIP
Lamb rump is a very lean meat. The fat in this recipe comes from the mayonnaise.

NIP
Energy   2723 kJ (651 Cal)
Total fat   30 g
Saturated fat   10 g
Carbohydrate   36 g

YUZU AND GREEN CHILLI JERK CHICKEN

ADAM LIAW

4 skinless, boneless chicken breasts
or thighs

3 tbsp olive oil

MARINADE

1 tbsp dried thyme

1 tsp hot chilli powder

1 tsp dried sage, ground

1 tbsp blade of mace

½ tsp freshly grated nutmeg

½ tsp ground cinnamon

1 tsp freshly ground black pepper

1 tbsp garlic powder

2 tbsp onion powder

2 tbsp soy sauce

2 tbsp yuzu juice or lemon juice

2 tbsp orange juice

3 large green chillies, thinly sliced

2 tbsp malt vinegar

2 tbsp white vinegar

lemon and lime cheeks, to serve

SERVES 4

Between two pieces of plastic wrap, beat chicken portions until they are a uniform thickness of about 1–2 cm (½–¾ in).

Mix together marinade ingredients, then whisk in oil until an emulsified dressing is formed.

Marinate chicken for at least 1 hour, preferably overnight.

Grill (broil) or barbecue chicken over high heat for a few minutes, basting well with any reserved marinade, until chicken is almost cooked through and any chilli covering the meat is blackened. Rest for a minute or two and serve immediately with lemon and lime cheeks (the chicken will continue to cook while off the heat).

NOTE: This marinade also works well for roasted whole chicken or grilled pork.

DIETITIAN TIP
This is a great low-fat way to prepare a tasty chicken dish.

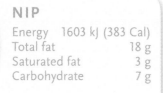

NIP
Energy   1603 kJ (383 Cal)
Total fat   18 g
Saturated fat   3 g
Carbohydrate   7 g

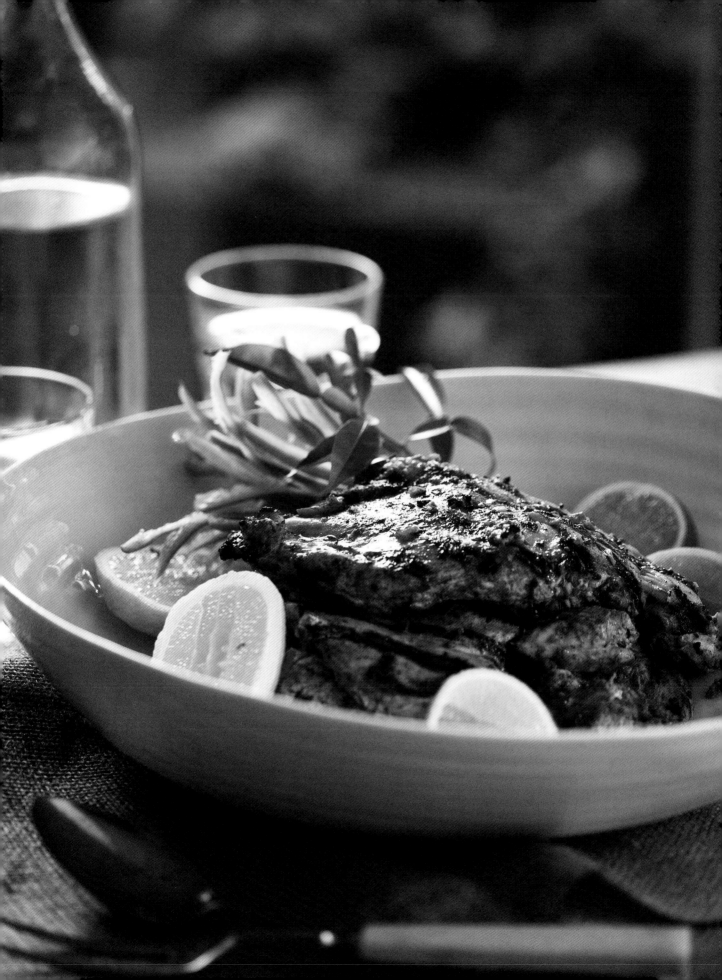

ROAST CHOOK WITH ROAST CARROT SALAD

MATT PRESTON

This is a simple low-carb take on the wonderful roast dinner combo of carrots and chook. Roasting gives all those delicious flavours of browning as well as intensifies the sweetness of your veg, while the witlof and vinegar add good fresh contrast to the dish. The nuts are there as much for crunch as to accent the chicken. Oh, and don't stress about serving this dish piping hot as I think it's actually nicer served warm — the flavours seem to jump out more.

1 tsp coriander (cilantro) seeds

½ tsp cumin seeds

sea salt

2 tbsp olive oil, plus 1½ tsp extra to grease roasting tin

4 boneless chicken breasts, skin on

2 leeks, white part only, sliced into 2-cm (¾-in) thick rounds

½ cup chicken stock or water

1 tbsp white wine vinegar

CARROT SALAD

16 finger-thick carrots, scrubbed

1 tbsp olive oil

sea salt and freshly ground black pepper

2 tbsp honey (optional) or good olive oil or whipped Greek-style yoghurt

1 witlof (chicory/Belgian endive), sliced crossways into strips

¼ red (Spanish) onion, finely chopped

200 g (7 oz) ricotta cheese

1 tbsp pistachio nuts, toasted

1 tbsp whole almonds, toasted

1 bunch dill, chopped

SERVES 4

Preheat oven to 180°C (350°F/Gas 4).

Crush coriander and cumin seeds together with a good pinch of salt. Mix with a good splash of olive oil and rub this into chicken breasts.

Oil a roasting tin, fill with sliced leeks and lay oiled chook breasts, skin side up, on top. Pour in chicken stock or water to keep the leeks moist. Bang in oven. The breasts will take about 45–55 minutes to cook, depending on how accurate your oven temperature gauge is. Cook chook under foil for the first 10 minutes, then cook for a further 15 minutes before checking. Basically, chook is ready when skin is golden and juices run clear when chook is pierced. When done, take chook breasts out to rest, covered. Place roasting tin on top of stove, sprinkle vinegar on leeks and give them a good stir, so vinegar sizzles in hot tin and you catch up all the delicious charry bits round corners of tin. Remove from heat and cover.

Meanwhile, for carrot salad, place carrots in a roasting tin, toss with olive oil, season well with salt and pepper and pop into oven. Roast for 45 minutes, with the chook, or until soft, almost caramelised and all roasty edged. Remove carrots from oven and transfer to a shallow bowl. Set aside to cool slightly.

Warm honey, if using, in a small saucepan over low heat. Remember that roasting will intensify carrots' sweetness anyway.

Now carrots are warm rather than hot, scatter witlof, onion and broken-up pieces of ricotta over top of them. Layer on nuts and drizzle with warmed honey. If you aren't using honey, drizzle on olive oil or yoghurt instead. Finally sprinkle on dill.

Serve this warm carrot salad with roast chicken breasts resting on a bed of sweet tangy roast leeks. Carbophiles can serve it with crusty warm bread.

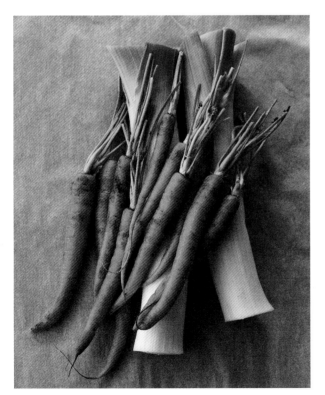

DIETITIAN TIP
You can remove the skin from the chicken to reduce the fat.

NIP
Includes honey

Energy	2479 kJ (592 Cal)
Total fat	29 g
Saturated fat	8 g
Carbohydrate	19 g

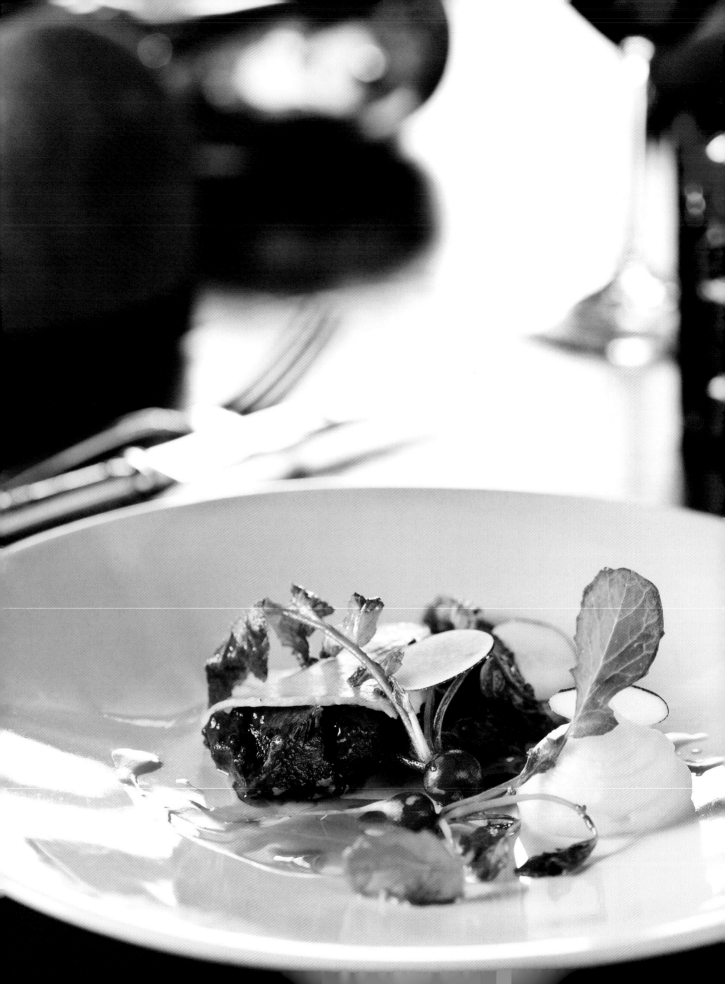

JOUE DE BOEUF, RADIS, ANETH

BEEF CHEEK, RADISH, DILL

SHANNON BENNETT

1 bunch red radishes

100 ml (3½ fl oz) grapeseed oil

BEEF CHEEKS

4 × 150 g (5½ oz) beef cheeks

200 g (7 oz) mirepoix (finely chopped celery, leek, carrot and onion)

4 cups (1 litre/35 fl oz) chicken stock

DILL OIL

1 bunch dill

1 cup (250 ml/9 fl oz) grapeseed oil

MILK SKIN

8 gelatine sheets

4 cups (1 litre/35 fl oz) milk

1 tbsp agar-agar

MASHED POTATO

2 sebago potatoes

125 g (4½ oz) butter, chopped into fine dice

1 tbsp warm milk, plus 1 tbsp extra, if necessary

1 tbsp sea salt

SERVES 4

Preheat oven to 95°C (200°F/Gas ½).

Keep beef cheeks whole, remove sinew and fat and reserve these off-cuts for sauce. Seal beef in a little grapeseed oil in a hot frying pan until golden brown. Remove from heat and place beef and mirepoix in a casserole dish. Cover with chicken stock, reserving the rest for the sauce. Braise in oven overnight or for 8 hours.

To make sauce, fry off beef trimmings in a saucepan, add reserved chicken stock and reduce until sauce coats the back of a spoon. Strain and keep warm over low heat until ready to serve.

To make dill oil, blanch dill in boiling water, refresh in iced water and pat dry with paper towel. Place in a food processor and blend with oil. Place in an airtight container and keep in fridge. Next day, strain through a fine sieve lined with muslin (cheesecloth) for 1 hour. Allow oil to strain slowly, do not force through.

To make milk skin, soak gelatine in cold water for 3 minutes and squeeze out excess water. Bring milk to the boil, whisk in agar-agar and remove from heat. Continue whisking for 1 minute. Stir in gelatine and strain into a deep tray, ensuring liquid reaches depth of 5 mm (¼ in). Cover with plastic wrap and place in fridge to set for 1 hour. Once set, cut into rectangular sheets about 10 × 9 cm (4 × 3½ in), or 25 g (1 oz) per portion.

Remove bigger leaves from radishes. Cut off bottom half of radish tops. Remove bigger radishes from stalks and set aside for crudités. Wash all leaves and radish bulbs vigorously to remove all sediment. For crisps, shallow-fry leaves in oil in a frying pan over medium heat until translucent and crispy, then drain on paper towel. For crudités, slice reserved radishes very thinly on a mandoline and store in iced water for 5 minutes. For tops, trim stalks and keep leaves looking natural.

To make mashed potato, cook potatoes for 25 minutes in salted boiling water. Test with a knife; they are cooked if the knife slides in without resistance. Immediately mash with 90 g (3¼ oz) butter through a food mill, then pass through a fine sieve. Mix in any visible butter with a wooden spoon. Place purée in a saucepan, add milk and whisk over low heat for 3–4 minutes. Add remaining butter, a quarter at a time, whisking rapidly. If the butter starts to separate, the purée is too hot. Remove from heat, beat in extra milk and whisk vigorously to bring it together. When all butter is incorporated, check seasoning and add salt if necessary.

Spoon mashed potato onto serving plates, then spoon on beef cheeks. Place radish tops, crisps and crudités randomly on plate to make it look as natural as possible. Place milk skin over cheeks and dress dish with dill oil. Spoon on sauce and serve.

DIETITIAN TIP
Beef cheeks are a high-fat part of the animal, so be careful with this type of meal if you are watching your weight.

NIP

Energy	2820 kJ (674 Cal)
Total fat	51 g
Saturated fat	23 g
Carbohydrate	17 g

SEARED BEEF FILLET, CHICKPEA, ROAST CHERRY TOMATO AND TREVISO SALAD WITH VINAIGRETTE

SEAN CORKERY

250 g (9 oz) truss cherry tomatoes

1 head treviso

1 baby cos (romaine) lettuce

150 g (5½ oz) cooked chickpeas

200 g (7 oz) beef fillet, thinly sliced

pinch of sea salt and freshly ground pepper

VINAIGRETTE

2 tsp lemon juice

2 tsp white wine vinegar

2 tsp white wine

100 ml (3½ fl oz) extra virgin olive oil

1 tbsp wholegrain mustard

SERVES 4

Preheat oven to 220°C (425°F/Gas 7).

Place cherry tomatoes in a roasting tin and roast for 5–10 minutes until skin starts to blister. Place in a bowl with treviso, cos and chickpeas.

Sear beef in a frying pan over high heat for about 45 seconds each side, keeping beef pink. Allow to rest for 5 minutes before slicing. Add to bowl with other salad ingredients.

For vinaigrette, whisk lemon juice, vinegar, white wine, olive oil and mustard in a small bowl until emulsified.

Lightly dress salad with vinaigrette, add salt and pepper and serve.

DIETITIAN TIP
Both a low-fat and a high-fibre meal.

NIP

Energy	1419 kJ (339 Cal)
Total fat	27 g
Saturated fat	5 g
Carbohydrate	8 g

JOUES DE BOEUF BOURGUIGNON

BEEF CHEEK BOURGUIGNON

MANU FEILDEL

I love to use beef cheek in this dish. It's such a gorgeous, rich cut that is just perfect for braising. This is one recipe that needs a good-quality red wine – a cheap 'cooking' wine changes the flavour completely and the dish truly suffers, so it's worth buying a great red wine. Just make sure you buy an extra bottle to drink with it.

1 onion, coarsely chopped

3 French shallots, coarsely chopped

2 carrots, coarsely chopped

2 garlic cloves, bruised

4 cups (1 litre/35 fl oz) red wine (burgundy or pinot noir)

1 thyme sprig

1 bay leaf

1 tsp black peppercorns

1.5 kg (3 lb 5 oz) beef cheeks, trimmed and connective tissue removed, cut into halves

1½ tbsp vegetable oil

60 g (2¼ oz) unsalted butter, chopped

sea salt

20 g (¾ oz) plain (all-purpose) flour

flat-leaf (Italian) parsley leaves, to serve (optional)

GARNISH

8 baby onions, peeled, root ends intact

large pinch of caster (superfine) sugar

30 g (1 oz) unsalted butter

sea salt and freshly ground pepper

1 × 200 g (7 oz) piece speck, cut into 3 × 1-cm (1¼ × ½-in) strips

2½ tbsp vegetable oil

400 g (14 oz) button mushrooms, wiped clean

SERVES 4

Place onion, shallot, carrot, garlic, red wine, thyme, bay leaf and peppercorns in a large bowl, add beef and combine well. Cover with plastic wrap and refrigerate overnight.

Remove meat from marinade and pat dry well with paper towel. Set aside. Strain marinade through a fine sieve into a large bowl and set aside; reserve vegetables and herbs.

Heat oil and butter in a large enamelled cast-iron casserole dish over medium–high heat. When butter begins to foam, cook meat in batches, seasoning it with salt as you go, for 8–10 minutes, or until golden all over. Remove from pan, reduce heat to low, then add reserved vegetables and herbs and stir for 6–8 minutes, or until light golden. Return meat to pan, sprinkle over flour and stir over low heat for 1 minute. Add reserved marinade, scraping pan to remove any cooked-on bits, and bring to the boil. Simmer, covered, for 2–3 hours, or until beef is tender, regularly skimming surface of any impurities. (The cooking time will vary, depending on the quality of the meat.)

Meanwhile, to make garnish, place onions, sugar, butter and a pinch of salt and pepper in a small saucepan. Add enough water to come halfway up side of onions, cover and cook over medium heat for 10 minutes. Cook, uncovered, for another 5 minutes, or until the water has evaporated and onions are tender and lightly coloured. Set aside. Heat a large frying pan over medium heat. Add speck and cook for 6–7 minutes, or until golden, then remove from pan and set aside. Add oil and, when hot, add mushrooms and season with salt and pepper. Toss for 5–6 minutes, or until golden and tender.

Drain meat and vegetables in a colander placed over a large bowl, then strain sauce through a fine sieve into a large saucepan. Use a ladle to remove fat from surface of sauce. Discard vegetables in colander. Add meat, glazed onions, mushrooms and speck to sauce. Simmer over low heat for 15 minutes, or until sauce has thickened and reduced. Check seasoning, add parsley, if desired, and serve.

This recipe is from *Manu's French Kitchen* by Manu Feildel (Penguin/Lantern, 2011).

DIETITIAN TIP
Beef cheeks are a higher fat meat — save for a special occasion if you are being careful with your energy and fat intake.

NIP

Energy	3553 kJ (849 Cal)
Total fat	53 g
Saturated fat	18 g
Carbohydrate	9 g

VITELLO TONNATO

GARY MEHIGAN

This classic Italian dish means perfectly pink, well seasoned veal and a smooth, delicate tuna sauce with a hint of anchovy and a kick of lemon and salty capers. Make it look pretty, with generous but restrained dollops of tuna sauce and a light drizzle of grassy extra virgin olive oil, finished with wafer-thin slices of lemon that you can eat but not squeeze. Bring me summer and a table in the sun.

1 × 450 g (1 lb) veal scotch fillet

6 cups (1.5 litres/52 fl oz) chicken stock or water

½ cup (120 g/4¼ oz) mayonnaise

6 anchovy fillets

3 tbsp large salted capers, rinsed and drained

130 g (4¾ oz) tinned tuna in oil, drained

finely grated zest and juice of ½ lemon

sea salt and freshly ground white pepper

1½ tbsp extra virgin olive oil

1 lemon, very thinly sliced

SERVES 4

Tie veal neatly with kitchen twine to hold its shape. Place veal in a saucepan and cover with chicken stock or water. Bring to the boil over high heat, then reduce heat to low and simmer for 35 minutes. To test if veal is ready, insert a meat thermometer into centre – it should register 48°C (118°F) for medium-done. Or insert a metal skewer, then place it on your bottom lip; it should be just warm. Transfer veal to a plate and leave to cool for 1 hour. When cool, slice thinly and set aside.

Blend mayonnaise, 2 anchovies, 2 tablespoons capers, tuna, and lemon zest and juice in a food processor until creamy and smooth. Season with a pinch of salt and a few twists of pepper.

Spoon a little sauce onto a large plate and spread out. Place veal slices on top and spoon over a little more sauce. Drizzle with olive oil and scatter with remaining capers, anchovies and very thin lemon slices, then serve.

NOTES: Veal is a beautiful meat but you have to trust your butcher as what is often sold labelled as veal isn't. I like to use the scotch fillet and rib loin of veal. As veal comes from a young animal it doesn't have a lot of fat, so overcooking can result in dry meat.

Tying the veal with kitchen twine means that it holds its shape during cooking. It is also easier to carve evenly, which improves its presentation.

Soaking the salted capers in a good quantity of water will help soften their saltiness. For best results, lift the capers from the water, leaving the salt granules behind.

This recipe is from *Comfort Food* by Gary Mehigan (Penguin/Lantern, 2010).

DIETITIAN TIP
By using lean veal and adding very little fat, this is a great low-fat meal from Gary.

NIP	
Energy	1744 kJ (417 Cal)
Total fat	24 g
Saturated fat	4 g
Carbohydrate	11 g

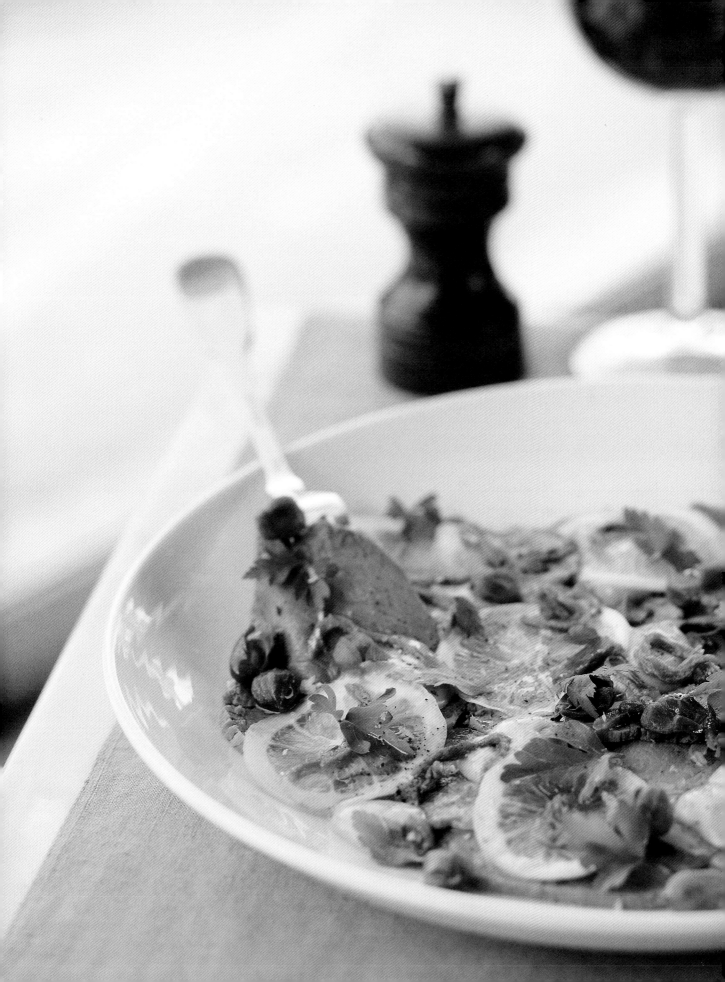

BARBECUED MARINATED CHICKEN WITH TABOULEH

NEIL PERRY

Easy to throw together and full of flavour, this marinade can be used on any meat or fish, and the tabouleh will be great as a side dish, or served on the plate. I often cook this dish at home, and love to serve it with a little seasoned yoghurt on top.

4 whole chicken legs, drumstick and thigh separated

extra virgin olive oil, for drizzling

1 lemon

freshly ground pepper

MARINADE

100 ml (3½ fl oz) extra virgin olive oil

4 garlic cloves

juice of ½ lemon

2 tsp ground coriander (cilantro)

2 tsp ground cumin

3 small red chillies, roughly chopped

3 thyme sprigs, leaves picked

sea salt

TABOULEH

heaped ¾ cup (140 g/5 oz) coarse burghul (bulgur)

2 vine-ripened tomatoes, peeled, seeds removed and chopped

1 Lebanese (short) cucumber, seeds removed and chopped

6 spring onions (scallions), chopped

½ bunch (about 75 g/2¾ oz) flat-leaf (Italian) parsley, stalks only, chopped

1 large handful flat-leaf (Italian) parsley leaves, roughly chopped

1 small handful mint leaves, roughly chopped

1 garlic clove, finely chopped

100 ml (3½ fl oz) extra virgin olive oil

juice of 1 lemon

sea salt and freshly ground pepper

SERVES 4

Process all marinade ingredients together until well combined.

Add chicken pieces to marinade, mix well and refrigerate for 2 hours.

Meanwhile, to make tabouleh, soak burghul in a bowl with enough water to cover for at least 1 hour. Drain and squeeze out excess water. Add remaining ingredients and mix well.

Heat a barbecue to hot, then place chicken on, skin side down. Cook for 5 minutes and turn, cook for a further 5 minutes then remove to a warm oven to rest for 5 minutes.

Spoon tabouleh onto each of four plates, and place a thigh and a drumstick on each plate. Drizzle with oil, squeeze over some lemon and add a generous grind of fresh pepper.

This recipe is from *Good Food* by Neil Perry (Murdoch Books, 2010).

DIETITIAN TIP
If you wish to make the fat content lower, be careful with the volume of marinade that you use.

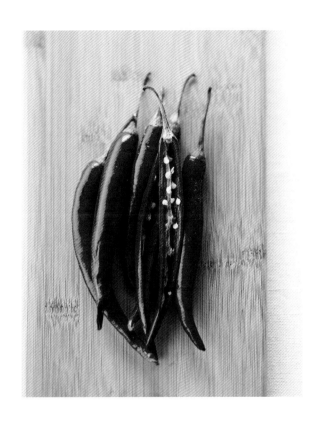

NIP
Energy   3390 kJ (810 Cal)
Total fat   59 g
Saturated fat   14 g
Carbohydrate   26 g

MOUNTAIN PEPPER LEAF WALLABY RUMP WITH BRAISED FENNEL AND APPLE

JENNICE KERSH AND RAYMOND KERSH

Kangaroo and wallaby are highly nutritious, full of iron and have .03 cholesterol, containing virtually no fat. It is important to remember that these meats should not be served well done; they should be juicy. Wallaby is very different from kangaroo in flavour and is quite subtle, not gamey. During the warmer months the braised fennel and apple is delicious served at room temperature.

4 × 80–110 g (2¾–3¾ oz) wallaby rumps or 2 × 200 g (7 oz) kangaroo rumps

1½ tbsp canola or olive oil

1 tsp mountain pepper leaf

coarsely chopped dill

BRAISED FENNEL AND APPLE

1 tbsp olive oil

1 large granny smith apple, peeled and cut into 5-mm (¼ -in) thick slices

½ large fennel bulb, cut into 1-cm (½ -in) thick slices

1 red (Spanish) onion, sliced into 2.5-mm (¹⁄₁₆-in) thick rings

1 large handful English spinach

1 garlic clove, chopped or smashed

3 tbsp white wine

3 tbsp water

sea salt and freshly ground pepper

SERVES 2

Preheat oven to 180°C (350°F/Gas 4).

Rub meat generously with canola oil and mountain pepper leaf, sear on both sides in a very hot ovenproof frying pan, reduce heat ever so slightly and cook for another 6 minutes. Place in oven for 6 minutes. Cover with foil and rest meat in a warm place for 3–4 minutes.

For braised fennel and apple, heat olive oil in a saucepan, add fruit and vegetable ingredients and garlic, and sauté quickly over medium–high heat, then add wine and water, cover with a lid and braise over medium heat for 10–12 minutes until tender, not overcooked.

To serve, place braised fennel and apple on dinner plates. Slice meat on an angle into three slices, then place on braised fennel and apple. Sprinkle dill over meat as a final touch.

NOTE: Ground mountain pepper leaf is available at Herbie's and The Essential Ingredient, both in Darling Street, Rozelle, Sydney. Some farmers' markets sell it, together with a good variety of other native herbs.

DIETITIAN TIP
By using wallaby or kangaroo, Jennice and Raymond have kept the fat content low but the flavour high.

NIP	
Energy	1957 kJ (468 Cal)
Total fat	27 g
Saturated fat	5 g
Carbohydrate	12 g

BRAISED SPATCHCOCK WITH OLIVES AND CAPERS

TETSUYA WAKUDA

2 × no. 5 spatchcocks (about 500 g/
1 lb 2 oz each), cut in half

sea salt and freshly ground pepper

2 cups (500 ml/17 fl oz) dry white wine

2 tbsp salted capers, rinsed

20 black olives

4 garlic cloves, finely chopped

2 tsp chopped oregano

100 ml (3½ fl oz) olive oil

1 tbsp finely chopped flat-leaf (Italian)
parsley

SERVES 4

Preheat oven to 200°C (400°F/Gas 6).

Place spatchcock halves, skin side up, in a roasting tin. Season with salt and pepper. Pour wine over each spatchcock until liquid reaches halfway up sides. Add water if more liquid is required. Add capers, olives, garlic and oregano to liquid. Drizzle olive oil over each spatchcock half and place in oven for 45 minutes, or until skin is golden and spatchcock is cooked through.

To serve, place a spatchcock half in the centre of each serving plate and spoon over a little braising liquid. Garnish with chopped parsley.

DIETITIAN TIP
Much of the alcohol will evaporate during the cooking process.

NIP
Energy   2332 kJ (557 Cal)
Total fat   40 g
Saturated fat   10 g
Carbohydrate   2 g

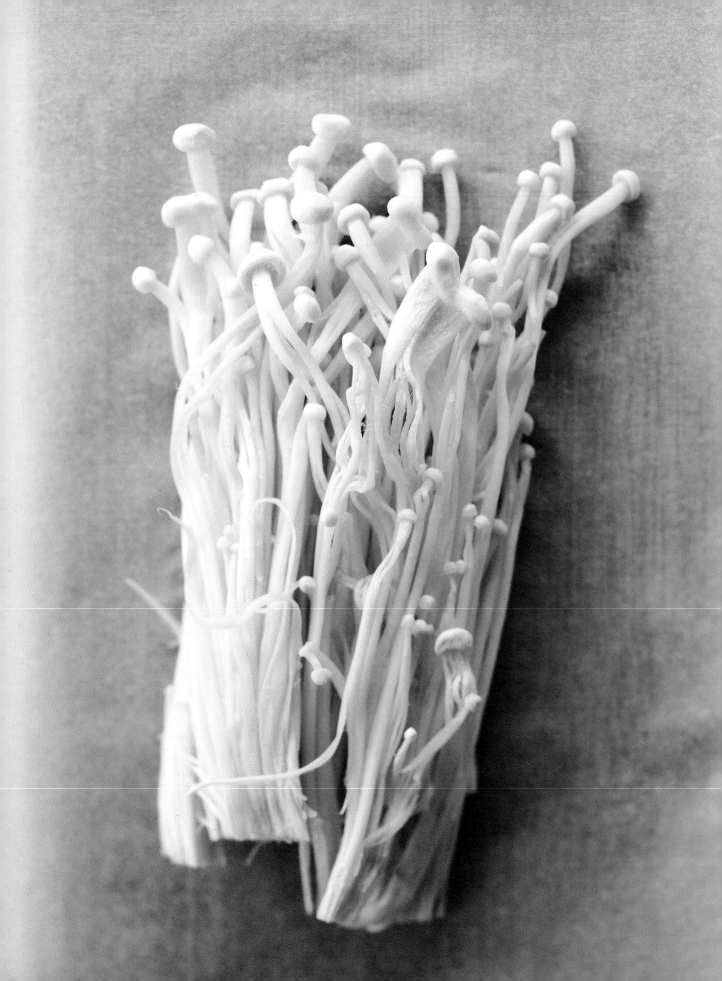